Speech in Action

of related interest

Speak, Move, Play and Learn with Children on the Autism Spectrum
Activities to Boost Communication Skills, Sensory Integration and
Coordination Using Simple Ideas from Speech and Language
Pathology and Occupational Therapy
Lois Jean Brady, America X Gonzalez, Maciej Zawadzki and Corinda Presley
Illustrated by Byron Roy James
ISBN 978 1 84905 872 8
eISBN 978 0 85700 531 1

Mouth and Tongue Let's Have Some Fun!
Karina Hopper
ISBN 978 1 84905 161 3
eISBN 978 0 85700 413 0

Rising to New Heights of Communication and Learning for Children with
Autism
The Definitive Guide to Using Alternative-Augmentative
Communication, Visual Strategies, and Learning Supports at Home
and School
Carol L. Spears and Vicki L. Turner
ISBN 978 1 84905 837 7
eISBN 978 0 85700 332 4

Challenge Me! (TM)
Speech and Communication Cards
Amanda Elliott
ISBN 978 1 84310 946 4

Attention and Listening in the Early Years
Sharon Garforth
ISBN 978 1 84905 024 1
eISBN 978 1 84642 958 3

Creative Expression Activities for Teens
Exploring Identity through Art, Craft and Journaling
Bonnie Thomas
ISBN 978 1 84905 842 1
eISBN 978 0 85700 417 8

Helping Children to Improve their Communication Skills
Therapeutic Activities for Teachers, Parents and Therapists
Deborah M. Plummer
Illustrated by Alice Harper
ISBN 978 1 84310 959 4
eISBN 978 0 85700 502 1

AMERICA X GONZALEZ, LOIS JEAN BRADY AND JIM ELLIOTT

Speech in Action

Interactive Activities Combining Speech Language Pathology and Adaptive Physical Education

Illustrated by Byron Roy James

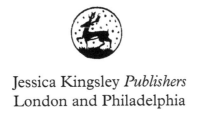

Jessica Kingsley *Publishers*
London and Philadelphia

'American Sign Language alphabet' diagram on p.137 is reproduced by permission of Martin Frost.

First published in 2011
by Jessica Kingsley Publishers
116 Pentonville Road
London N1 9JB, UK
and
400 Market Street, Suite 400
Philadelphia, PA 19106, USA

www.jkp.com

Library of Congress Cataloging in Publication Data
Gonzalez, America X.
  Speech in action : interactive activities combining speech language pathology with adaptive physical education / America X Gonzalez, Lois Jean Brady and Jim Elliott ; illustrated by Byron Roy James.
      p. cm.
  Includes bibliographical references.
  ISBN 978-1-84905-846-9 (alk. paper)
 1. Speech therapy. 2. Language disorders--Treatment . 3. Physical education and training. 4. Autism spectrum disorders I. Brady, Lois Jean. II. Elliott, Jim. III. Title.
  RC423.G665 2011
  616.85'506--dc22
                                                                              2010030183

British Library Cataloguing in Publication Data
A CIP catalogue record for this book is available from the British Library

ISBN 978 1 84905 846 9
eISBN 978 0 85700 500 7

To all of our students,
whose enthusiasm and warm smiles
have pushed us to be better.

ACKNOWLEDGMENTS

Jeani's

I would like to give a super special thank-you to Gary for being my gardener, housekeeper, babysitter, cook, and driver while I spent many long hours tapping at the keyboard and mumbling at the ceiling. A special thanks to my mom who is still my biggest fan and heartiest supporter. Also, I would like to recognize my children Ian and Stephanie who finally learned to do their homework and clean their rooms by themselves. Many heartfelt thanks to Helen Ibbotson, Rachel Menzies, and everyone at Jessica Kingsley Publishers who was involved in the publication of this book. However, the individuals who deserve the most acknowledgments are the students and participants themselves. You are the models, the guides that cemented the principles of this book. Without your participation, the theory that movement enhances language would be just that, a theory. You brought it to life and showed me a new paradigm to conduct therapy and remediation that truly works. Now I can share it with the rest of the world. Thank you!

Jim's

I would like to acknowledge my family for supporting me on this project. I also would like to thank the staff and students for their support and input on this project.

America's

I'd like to acknowledge my beautiful family for all of their support and encouragement throughout this process. If it weren't for the unending love and respect that I received from my mother and my father I don't think that I would have been the same person I am today. I'd also like to thank my sister Citlalli for her wonderful insight, and my brothers Daniel, Jose, Carlos, and Ricky for their relentless jokes, mostly at my expense. Without laughter there is no light. My gratitude extends to Larry for being my best friend and confidant for all these years and also to the staff and students whom I have had the privilege of working with. Thank you all for the wonderful memories.

CONTENTS

ABOUT THE ILLUSTRATOR

Byron Roy James came into this world early, at three pounds in a rural Russian hospital, where he stayed for his first 15 months. He was adopted by American parents whom Byron made very proud and happy. Byron's talents presented themselves quickly, one of them being his artwork. His specialty was drawing in three-dimensional perspectives at the age of five without any instruction. Byron has never stopped drawing. His parents discovered his Asperger gifts and challenges early, and Byron has grown into a healthy, fun-loving, kind, talented, and social young man. Currently, Byron is pursuing his varied interests and hobbies of cooking, drawing cityscapes, studying modern transportation systems, road biking, racquetball, turtles, and just having a good time with family. He lives in Pleasant Hill, California, with his parents, his 12-year-old brother and sister, and a menagerie of family pets. He'll be entering high school in the fall.

INTRODUCTION

What is Speech in Action?

Speech language pathologists, sometimes called speech therapists, assess, diagnose, treat, and help to prevent disorders related to speech, language, cognitive-communication, voice, swallowing, and fluency (Bureau of Labor Statistics 2010). Adapted physical education has been described as:

> the art and science of developing and implementing a carefully designed physical education instructional program for an individual with a disability, based on a comprehensive assessment, to give the individual the skills necessary for a lifetime of rich leisure, recreation, and sport experiences (Auxter *et al.* 2009).

Speech in Action is the combination of speech pathology and adaptive physical education (APE) merging harmoniously in a multimodality therapy session. This idea was born from a collaborative effort between three members of a designated instructional services team as we were trying to figure out how to best serve our clients. We began forming lesson plans that integrated speech theories and physical education curriculum while still maintaining a high interest in the material from our students.

Jeani Brady, SLP; America X Gonzalez, SLPA; and Jim Elliott, APE, have combined nearly five decades of hands-on experience with autistic spectrum disorders and developmentally disabled children and adults. For the past five years we have worked together and focused on students who have been diagnosed with autism, Asperger's syndrome, Down's syndrome, and severe emotional distress. We began writing lesson plans to encourage and enhance language acquisition and movement while making the experience more engaging for our students. Our clients have not only met their goals but look forward to every session because they truly appreciate the exciting games and techniques we have created. Speech in Action makes learning an unforgettable experience that has our students asking for more time and volunteering to work with us.

Why it works

Traditional education has relied on treating the brain and the body as if they were made up of separate components. Some educators believe that these separate components comprise one section for music, one for art, one for physical education, one for math, and another for language. That is the main reason why we teach academic subjects in isolation from one another in our schools. This separation of our attributes seems unnecessary considering the brain is a multi-function parallel processor. It can take in information at many different levels simultaneously and process the information in different ways instantaneously (Jensen 2000). Taking the idea that the whole is better than the sum of all parts we can begin to understand why Speech in Action's synergistic approach can yield better results than simply doing these therapies in isolation.

Researchers have been studying the effects of physical activity on speech and language development for some time now. There has been resounding evidence that by incorporating language with physical movement students can develop language in higher proportions than if they had a language lesson without adding the physical component. Research suggests that physical activity integration may help communication skills for any student, including those with special needs (e.g. Jobling, Birji-Babul, and Nichols 2006; Waugh, Bowers, and French 2007). Even simple movements such as tapping have been found to have an effect on learning language. It is important to use the hands to integrate physicality into a lesson. For instance, tapping rhythms makes learning more effective by encouraging a "hands-on" approach to learning and by stimulating different parts of the brain. Using movement and rhythm stimulates the frontal lobes of the brain and also enriches language and the development of motor skills (Brewer and Campbell 1991). It should come as no surprise that clapping along to a song or using body movements prevail in childhood games and music like "My Dog Bingo"; "Head, Shoulders, Knees, and Toes"; "Pat-a-Cake"; "I'm a Little Teapot"; "The Wheels on the Bus"; "Hokey Pokey"; and "Here We Go Loopty Loo." These songs and games are taught at a very early age even to children who are just learning to speak. For children who cannot yet respond verbally or who have no language ability, movement becomes the mode of expression. Children learn to express themselves and are inadvertently activating the vestibular system (an ear element responsible for balance and movement), which needs to be activated in order for learning to take place (Hannaford 1995).

According to Hannaford, human beings learn 10 percent of what they read, 20 percent of what they hear, 30 percent of what they see, 50 percent of what they see and hear, 70 percent of what is discussed, 80 percent of what is experienced, and 95 percent of what is actively taught (Hannaford 1995). It is clear that human brains learn more when they are experiencing the world instead of merely reading or hearing about it. But much of today's education centers on teaching through reading out of books in the classroom or listening to lectures. As Jensen states:

> The result is bored or frustrated learners who then perpetuate the underachievement cycle. What this means to learning is that we understand complex topics better when we experience them with rich sensory input, as opposed to merely reading or hearing about the subject (2000, pp. 3, 12, 13).

If we were to pick the top two ways of learning then experiencing and actively teaching would win. The similarities between these two are that they are the modalities that encourage the use of most of our senses at one time. That is why Speech in Action is so effective, because we use the synergistic approach to learning and we strive to engage as much of the brain at once as we can so learning can be optimized.

According to Kovar *et al.* (2007) it is important to encourage physical movement because it will help kids stay healthy. With today's scary statistics about childhood obesity we can see how a program like Speech in Action can have many levels of benefits. The authors also suggested that physical movement stimulates brain activity to improve learning. In addition,

> as students develop physically, they can better develop mentally. For example, if a student cannot skip then that same student probably cannot read, because physical and cognitive development works together. Speech faculty make their students stand up to give speeches, gesture to add meaning, and join together for group problem solving. Speech teachers have used physical activities to teach nonverbal communication long before the strategy was popular in other fields (Herman and Kirschenbaum 1990).

Communication and physical activity go together.

How it works

Speech in Action works by using the natural design of games. By using movement and social interactions, which are already present in the scheme of sports and teamwork, one can get maximum results for learning.

Cooperative game structure with young children has generally been found to be beneficial in promoting pro-social behavior. Play has many beneficial effects on the development of social skills in young children (Hill and Reed 1990). In this manner we can take an already existing ideology and reap its benefits without boring the children. The reason we can enhance communication skills in the movement setting is because children tend to find this environment very rewarding and exciting.

Teaching social pragmatics during a physical activity is easy to do since the internal structures of most games are built with these unwritten rules within them. For example, even the most solitary game like golf still requires that the player take turns at the tee, that there be no interruption by another player while hitting the ball, that the player in the lead not gloat, that the winner not over-celebrate, and that if one makes a mistake that we not make fun of them or if it is our mistake that we not throw a tantrum. These unwritten laws are what make up our social pragmatics. Many believe that playing sports and games alone cannot teach social skills. The nature of the experience and instruction, however, are what is critical to the learning of social skills (Gould 1987). When we do Speech in Action we are giving our students the opportunity to learn invaluable lessons in social interactions while reinforcing the lessons with a physical action that will cement the lessons into their brains.

Who should do Speech in Action?

Everyone! Even though the lesson plans were originally created with special education students in mind, we soon found out that these lessons could prove very helpful for mainstreamed children from preschool through elementary. The lessons seem to attract the attention of all our students alike. Some games are designed with specific populations, and the chapters are divided so that you can quickly and easily locate your target group and then find a ton of fun activities to do. The chapters are divided into warm-up activities; beginning level for lower-functioning students; intermediate level for moderately higher goals; and advanced level for abstract thought, figurative language, multiple meanings, idioms, and advanced physical exercises.

According to DiCarlo, Banajee, and Stricklin, "Children with speech and language delays or those who are nonverbal as a result of a particular disability or multiple disabilities might use augmentative or alternative systems to communicate" (2000, pp.3 and 18–26). Zittel adds that:

Young children with autism often have very sophisticated picture systems in place to assist with identifying activities, equipment, activity directions, and transitions. Having a child understand *what to do* and *when to do it* often decreases the time needed to manage unwanted behaviors" (2005, p.391).

By having picture-system elements spread about the therapy room and across settings the student will be more engaged in making requests while integrating the language component of the physical activity in the movement environment.

Where should I do Speech in Action?

Everywhere! The great advantage of the Speech in Action lessons is that they were designed with flexibility and portability in mind. The main purpose is to make it so that therapists and nonprofessionals alike can do these activities with relative ease. We have suggested items to use for the activities like a ball or a hoop, but these can easily be made out of crumpled newspaper held together with tape and a wastebasket or empty box. The idea is to use and reuse items readily available to you. By recycling things around the house or school for the activities we help to keep our mother earth clean.

The ideal setting for developing speech and language is a physical education setting (Connor-Kuntz and Dummer 1996). However, any place where movement won't be hindered is an ideal location for Speech in Action. Researchers believe that "social development in physical education classes present situations in which young people are required to interact with each other . . . in a way that is different from the standard academic environment" (Mutrie 1997). In fact, if students interact with one another in the regular academic setting they will often be either punished for talking in class or accused of cheating. That is why it is imperative that we take advantage of the few social situations left in school to teach language, and what better way to do that than with Speech in Action.

Another great advantage of Speech in Action is that the portability of the lessons allows for a freedom to roam around the real-world environment. By interacting with the world, students can experience the knowledge they are learning first hand and can then generalize the themes from the lessons immediately. Generalization is important because it means that a child is putting the information they learned to practical use, and in the end that is what we want them to do—to apply what they learned and thrive in the world around them.

HOW TO USE THIS BOOK

This book was made with the thought of relative ease in mind. It is put together in a way that enables the user to open up the book to any page and be able to find a fun activity that can be done with a minimal number of materials and with tons of variations to adjust to the appropriate level of the child involved. Most of the lesson plans have materials that will be readily available in the home, school, and therapy room. There are even some variations that can be done with no materials at all. The practicality of the lesson plans was purposefully made a priority in order to reach out to busy parents, therapists, day-care providers, and schoolteachers. In a world that seems to always be on the run and constantly rushing, a simple yet effective book can be a valuable tool in our quest for educating our young.

We have purposefully kept the materials used in this book simple and readily available to everyone so that these activities can be utilized in the home, school, and community environments. By reinforcing the lessons we are providing our children with more opportunities to practice the lesson and increasing the chances that they will remember what we taught. Inter-environmental generalization promotes fluidity and connectivity.

In the book we will use terms like *teacher*, *student*, *child*, and *group*. A *group* can be a parent and child, or a parent and a few children, or a therapist and one or more clients. Day-care providers and their students can also be put under the term *group* as it applies in this book. Keep in mind, however, that the term *teacher* is interchangeable for parents, day-care providers, and therapists alike. After all, anyone who teaches a lesson is a teacher even if they are also a parent. The reasoning behind this train of thought is that parents teach their children, care providers teach their students, and therapists teach their clients. We are all teachers and we are all in this together. That is why we chose to come together to bridge the gap of educational systems now in place and to put our collaborative efforts forward in an attempt to reach out to our children in a way that inspires them to learn.

HOW TO PRAISE YOUR STUDENT AND ENCOURAGE HEALTHY SELF-ESTEEM

There are numerous ways to praise someone, but some are more successful than others. The subject of praising others has gotten a lot of attention in the past ten years. Most teachers seem to be content with praise that is easy to dole out and that shows the emphasis on the actual praise rather than on the achievement. Terms like "Awesome," "Great," "Amazing," and "Give me five" are in this category. They are centered around the way that the praise makes a child feel rather than praising the individual achievement. In child development circles practitioners have started to get away from the use of empty praise and have moved toward a more specific and bias-neutral praise agenda. The praise should also refrain from making assumptions. When praising anyone make sure to always commend the effort. The long hours gathering the research should be praised more than the grade on the research paper. And finally, try to praise physical qualities carefully. In fact they should be mostly avoided because the praise should be about things the child has achieved or attained, and more often than not physical characteristics cannot be changed. Here are a few examples of what to say and what not to say.

Praise should be specific

By praising the exact accomplishment we can make children more aware of their true gifts. When you tell children why they did something good they will be more likely to understand exactly what they did right and will be more likely to repeat it. It will also help them learn more about their identity if they begin to learn at an early age what exactly they are good at and what they need to work on.

Vague Praise	Specific Praise
Awesome!	Awesome way of staying inside the lines!
Great job!	Great color scheme!
Amazing work!	Amazing details and perspective!
You have a cool project! We all liked it.	I like the way your project got our attention with all the lights and sounds.

Praise should not be biased

We are in world that has a huge variety of social norms and gender roles that play a part in our development. Some of these norms or roles have changed with the passage of time. As teachers and parents we have a responsibility to our children that enables us to shape their little minds. Sometimes we might inadvertently propagate these roles and norms but we must be careful not to bias our children. We should let the children explore the world around them without limiting their choices.

Biased Praise	Biased Outcome	Unbiased Praise	Unbiased Outcome
You look so pretty today!	Might feel like she wasn't pretty before.	Wow, you are wearing a new hairdo today!	Might feel praised and she got some positive attention.
You are such a strong boy!	Propagates the role of the strong boy and weak girl.	You carried the books all by yourself!	Promotes independence.
You are so smart!	Might make a child shy away from trying things he is not good at later in life.	You finished the project first! It must have been easy for you.	Might want to challenge himself to do things that will be harder next time.

Praise should not make assumptions

When we see a child's drawing or ceramic sculpture we often feel compelled to explain the art in terms that are familiar to us. But we have to realize that children have their own way of seeing the world. So that drawing of a whale-looking thing in the ocean might be an airplane inside a cloud. Children look to us for guidance and to explain the world to them. Unfortunately, we unnecessarily impose our expectations on children when it comes to art, feelings, music, and the endless ways that they express themselves. This is a good time to realize that children are expressing themselves to us. It is our turn to listen to what they have created, and we must not put ourselves in their work.

I have seen teachers tell their kids that flowers can't grow on the roof of a house, that pigs don't belong inside the house, and that there can't be a moon and a sun in the sky at the same time. But I have also seen all these scenarios in real life. My uncle's cottage has flowers and moss growing on the roof, my friend has a pig that lives with her, and I have seen the moon out when it is daytime. So we have to check ourselves and make sure we don't impose our views on the child's art. Praise in this area requires that we praise the specific concepts and contents in a way that does not denote an assumption on our behalf. We shouldn't, however, ask, "What is this?" because it might not be anything at all. If a teacher asks a child who just drew something, "That looks great. What is it?" then the child might feel pressure to make up something even though he might not have drawn anything in particular. He might feel like we are expecting him to draw something concrete. But in fact he might have just been drawing random lines because the crayon felt good as it slid on the paper or because he liked the way the colors blended together. The best thing to do is to ask the child to explain what he did. In this way we do not have to make assumptions and the child won't feel a need to meet our expectations from those assumptions.

Praise with Assumptions	Outcome of Assumptions	Praise without Assumptions	Outcome of Not Assuming
Those are some pretty cows in the field!	The drawings might not be cows. They could be horses or goats, robots, imaginary unicorns, etc.	I like the way your picture turned out. Can you explain what you drew to me?	We find out exactly what they drew. (The drawings might have just been random shapes.)
His clothes are red so it must be Santa Claus! Good job!	Children might assume that things have to be done in a certain way and won't explore their creativity.	I like this red object.	The child will receive the praise and might feel compelled to give you a verbal interpretation of his or her drawing.

CHAPTER 1

Warm-Ups, Cool-Downs, and Breathing

Time spent on warming up and cooling down is time well spent. Warm-ups, cool-downs, and proper breathing can energize the brain, help prevent injury, and reduce muscle soreness. Warming up can prepare your body, muscles, brain, and heart for a physical activity. Cooling down can help bring your heart rate back to normal and prepare your muscles for the next time you are active. Warm-up, cool-down, and breathing activities should be five to ten minutes in duration. Warm-up activities are typically slightly more vigorous than cool-down activities.

Proper respiration is a key factor in enhancing communication disorders. Breathing exercises not only teach proper respiration but also benefit the student by promoting relaxation, oxygenating the blood, increasing concentration, and strengthening the central nervous system.

From the point of view of the speech pathologist, breath is the basis of speech. All sounds, words, and sentences begin with airflow (breath).

Stretching is important for a good warm-up and cool-down and it is one of the best ways to prevent and avoid soreness, cramps, and injury. Stretching is important for the whole body, including oral and facial muscles.

Benefits of warming up

- It increases the speed of contraction and relaxation of muscles.
- It decreases high tone and increases low tone.
- More oxygen is utilized at higher muscle temperatures.
- It increases the blood flow to active tissue.
- It allows for a controlled heart rate increase.

- It allows the student to mentally focus.
- It increases range of motion and flexibility.
- It increases sensory regulation.
- It builds confidence.

Benefits of cooling down

- It aids in ridding the body of waste products.
- It reduces the chance of dizziness or fainting.
- It reduces the level of adrenaline in the blood.
- It allows the heart rate to return to resting.

One last word: Be kind to yourself. Go slowly, especially in the beginning. Pushing yourself too hard may cause injury and you won't enjoy the activity.

Deep Breath Stretch

Purpose: This is an excellent beginning and ending exercise. Encourage students to breathe during the day to self-regulate. Breathing promotes self- and body awareness, balance, concentration, and focus and it improves sensory regulation. It prepares the body for physical and psychological exercises. Students will learn to use similes to express what their bodies are doing.

Materials: Calming music.

Description: Have the students stand facing you. The students should stand tall and strong like a mountain with feet slightly apart. Rock slightly back and forth on your feet to plant them like the roots of a tree.

- Observe your own natural breath.

- Watch as your abdomen rises and then falls.

- Only let the abdomen rise and fall; keep the chest still. (Some students may need to put their hand on their abdomen for visual feedback.)

- Now deepen, lengthen, and extend that movement while inhaling five to ten times.

- Add arm movements:

  ○ Inhale as you raise your arms to the sky like a (have students fill in).

  ○ Exhale slowly and lower your arms like a (have students fill in).

Variations:

1. The students can lie on the floor like a snake and make hissing sounds while breathing.

2. In the lying position, they can put a light book on their abdomen and watch it rise and fall with each breath. Breathe for several minutes with eyes closed. This is an excellent activity to do at the end of a session to calm the body and relieve stress and anxiety.

WARM-UPS, COOL-DOWNS, AND BREATHING

23

The Cobra

Purpose: This traditional yoga activity will stretch and strengthen back and arm muscles. This activity will increase the ability to follow multistep directions, breath support for speech, body awareness, and body-part identification.

Materials: Quiet to moderate tempo music if available.

Description: Students follow you through a series of exercises and stretches.

- Lie down on your stomach with legs together, elbows bent, and hands by your chest (see the illustration).

- Slowly take a deep breath and raise your head and chest up from the floor as high as they will go. Use your arms as supports, like a cobra in striking position.

- Take two to three deep breaths.

- Lower your chest back to the floor.

- Repeat five to ten times.

- Hips should not leave the floor.

Variations:

1. When taking a deep breath, hiss and stick your tongue out like a snake to modulate airflow.

2. When your chest is raised off the floor, try to touch the top of your head with your toes. Hold and release.

3. Raise your chest and legs off the floor as far as possible and hold your arms in front of you (like Superman). Hold your breath and release five to ten times.

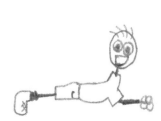 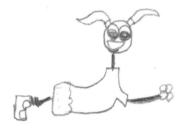

The cobra

Snow Angel Stretch

Purpose: This activity will increase strength and range of motion for leg, arm, and trunk muscles. It will develop flexibility, receptive language skills, body awareness, and body-part identification. And it encourages imagination!

Materials: Music can be used to enhance this activity.

Description: You verbally guide the students through a series of movements and encourage them to use their imagination.

- Students lie on the floor or mats, if available, with arms and legs stretched as if someone were pulling on them.

- You will encourage the students to imagine that they are snow angels and can fly by slowly moving their wings and legs in and out and up and down (like a jumping jack).

- Now imagine a wind comes and blows your wings and legs to one side. The students can take deep breaths and blow like the wind. Stop the wind by flexing your hands and feet.

- Now the wind is blowing from the other side. The students again take a deep breath and blow like the wind. Stop the wind by flexing your hands and feet.

- Oh, no! Now the wind is blowing your wings to the opposite side of your legs and vice versa. The students can blow like the wind. Stop the wind by flexing your hands and feet.

- It's beginning to snow! Stretch your wings and legs into the air to catch the snow.

Variations:

1. The students can imagine they are starfish and the water and waves are moving their arms, legs, and rays (the arms of a starfish) instead of the wind. They can make whooshing sounds for the ocean.

2. While lying on their backs, the students can pretend to be a spider walking on the ceiling, ride an invisible bicycle, or simply touch their hand to the opposite foot depending on the age of the student.

WARM-UPS, COOL-DOWNS, AND BREATHING

25

Compliment Circle

Purpose: This activity can be used as a cool-down or warm-up exercise. It promotes stretching, gross motor skills, good manners, turn taking, pragmatic skills, and diplomacy.

Materials: Each individual will need a bottle, a pencil, a pen, or any object that can be used as a pointer. Background music is welcome.

Description: The students and you sit in a circle with legs stretched in a V position. Each student places their pointer as far to the middle of the circle as they can. Everyone sits up straight and touches their object five times alternating left and right hands. On the fifth touch, the students will spin their pointers. They will then take turns complimenting the person their pointer is pointing at. If the pointer is pointing at them, they will give a self-compliment. After everyone has given a compliment, the pointers are moved one inch (two centimeters) farther away and the routine begins again.

Variations:

1. Use greetings instead of compliments as a warm-up activity.

2. Use salutations in a cool-down, goodbye activity.

The Warrior

Purpose: This traditional yoga pose improves balance, concentration, ability to follow multistep directions, body awareness, and sensory integration—and it's fun. Targeted language concepts are front, back, up, down, slow, slower, forward, left, right, bend, and straight.

Materials: Music is great, if available, at a quiet to moderate tempo.

Description: Students should follow you through the series of steps.

- Students should stand strong like a tree and take a few deep breaths.
- Step out with the right foot about four feet (one meter) and turn the left foot outward.
- Bend your right knee until it is above your ankle.
- Raise your arms over your head.
- Slowly lower your arms until the right arm is facing to the front and the left is facing to the back (like shooting an arrow).
- Take two to three deep breaths.
- Lower your arms and bring your legs together.
- Repeat with the left leg lunging and left arm reaching to the front.

Variations:

1. While you are in warrior pose and your arms are stretching to the front and back, slowly turn your trunk until your arms are pointing the opposite way.

2. While your arms are raised up over your head, do ten warriors—lunging steps around the room—then stop and slowly lower your arms and bring your feet together.

Oral Motor Stretches

Purpose: This activity prepares oral motor muscles and structures for activities, stretching, and increased range of motion.

Materials: None.

Description: The students follow you through a series of exercises and stretches.

- The students slowly turn their heads left, right, forward, and backward.

- They move their heads in large slow circles.

- They open their mouths wide and close them tightly in a pucker.

- They exaggerate and alternate the *ooo* and *eee* sounds (pretend they are animals).

- They close their eyes tight, scrunch their faces, and count to three.

- They open their eyes and mouths wide as if surprised.

- They rotate the tongue around the inside of their mouths, pushing slightly on their cheeks and lips as they go around (tongue sweep).

Variations:

1. Students may use their hands and arms to help exaggerate movements and stretch the entire upper body.

2. Syllables (consonant–vowel, CV) can be used to the beat of music (*la la la, da da da, ma ma ma, pa pa pa, me mu ma*).

3. Clicking, clucking, raspberries, smacking, blowing kisses, and other sounds can be used as warm-ups.

Facial Stretches

Purpose: This activity will increase students' ability to interpret and display facial expressions and body language. It will improve muscle tone, range of motion, and strength for articulators.

Materials: Music can be used to enhance the activity if available.

Description: Have the students stand in a circle so that they can see one another. You may demonstrate or have a picture of an emotion. The students are to exaggerate the emotion on their faces and with body language. Don't forget to have them use their tongues (e.g. raspberry or sticking it out as if at a bully).

Variations:

1. Have the students add sound effects with the facial expression.

2. They can walk, skip, limp, or crawl appropriate to the emotion.

3. You can ask for faces only or bodies only.

4. If mirrors are available the students can observe themselves, or they can partner up and take turns using each other as the mirror.

Know Your Body Parts

Purpose: This activity will increase body awareness and identification, stretch muscles and increase range of motion, encourage group participation, and enhance the ability to follow multistep directions.

Materials: In this activity you will need pictures of body parts (human or animal, see the "Table of body parts" in the Appendix for some ideas) that are put together on a poster, wall, or sheet of cardboard and attached with Velcro™, felt, or sticky dots. Be sure to include the song "Head, Shoulders, Knees, and Toes" at the end of the activity.

Description: At the beginning of the activity, the students and you will choose a body part by touching or taking the part desired from the board. After choices have been made, they all sit or stand in a circle. Each person names and touches the body part they have chosen and signs or gestures should be incorporated. You will start by holding your body part up and saying, "I have an *arm*, what can you do with an *arm*?"

- Stretch high and low.
- Stretch arms forward and across midline.
- Make small, medium, and big circles.
- Shake and bend.
- Rub and squeeze.
- Twist and turn.

The next person in the circle takes their turn by holding up his or her body part and repeating the sequence. When all the students have had their turn, those who chose head, shoulder, knees, and toes move to the center and lead the song "Head, Shoulders, Knees, and Toes" while touching each part. When finished with the activity, they replace the pictures on the board in the correct positions.

Variations:

1. Students can use the names of bones to replace body parts. At the end of the activity they can sing "Dem Bones" (see "'Dem Bones' lyrics" in the Appendix) while touching each named part. You may want to replace some of the original words with the actual name of the bone, such as *head bone* with *cranium*.

Right to Left

Purpose: Right to Left promotes both midline movements that help brain hemispheres work together and body awareness; identification of body parts; balance; coordination; and identification of the concepts left, right, forward, and reverse.

Materials: Music can be used to enhance the activity.

Description: Students will follow you through a series of exercises and stretches.

- Raise your right hand and slowly move in large circles to the side and then in front of yourself. (Circles should be both forward and reverse.)
- Raise your left hand and slowly move in large circles to the side and then in front of yourself.
- Move both left and right together in the same manner to the side and in front of yourself.
- Reach with your right hand and touch your left toe and vice versa.
- Reach with your right elbow and touch your left knee and vice versa.
- Stand with your body still and turn your head right and left.
- Stand with your feet still and twist and turn your body left and right.
- Sit on the floor with your legs stretched out in a V and again touch your left hand to your right foot, your left elbow to your right knee, and vice versa.

Encourage the students to watch others if they have not mastered the concepts of left and right.

Variations:

1. Have the students pair up and use each other as a mirror image.
2. Include tongue, lips, and eyes.
3. Students can take turns leading or coleading the activity.
4. The activity can be done in a Simon-Says format.
5. If music is used, the pace can change to fit the student level and mood of activity.

31

Reach For ...

Purpose: To develop flexibility by having the students stretch and to develop language concepts of categorization, descriptions, and imagination.

Materials: Room to move; exercise ball (optional).

Description: Clear enough space so that each student can have room to stretch without bumping into anything. Have the students sit on an exercise ball, chair, curb, or floor. Ask them each what they want to reach for, or give them a category (things in a tree, things on a shelf, things on your shoe, etc.). Then have them do the stretch upward, sideways, or downward. For instance, when stretching your hands up say, "I am reaching up toward the stars" and when stretching downward say, "I am reaching for my shoes." Have the students get creative so that they may increase their expressive vocabulary. Some interesting answers I have received for a downward stretch have been, "Reach down for the microbes," "molecules of dirt," "atoms," and "bugs."

Variations:

1. If you don't have exercise balls then you could always do regular stretches by standing upright or sitting on the floor. Have the students reach for things in their surroundings if they are younger (cabinets, shelves, or trees if outside), and have them reach for abstract things if they are older so the game stays interesting (air, Japan, cardinal points, etc.).

Listen

Purpose: This activity improves auditory processing, focus, attention, and the ability to give and follow directions. It targets gross muscle movement, coordination, and body awareness.

Materials: None.

Description: All participants can be standing or sitting in a loose circle. This activity begins with you demonstrating how to make different noises with the body, lips, and mouth. Everyone practices clapping, snapping, stomping, whistling, sneezing, popping their lips, and slapping their hands on the floor and their thighs. Once the students have practiced making sounds, explain that they are only going to listen and recreate the same sounds in the same sequence as the leader. All students should then either close their eyes or turn their backs to you. Clap once. All the students should clap once. Now clap then stomp. All students should clap then stomp. Then continue sequencing sounds (matching the students' ability level) for several minutes. The students can take turns being the leader.

Variations:

1. When the students have mastered listening in a quiet environment, add background music or noise. The music or noise can become louder and louder or your voice can become softer and softer to encourage better listening skills.

2. The leader can make noises to a beat or song (much like the musical STOMP).

3. Quiet gaps of five to ten seconds can be integrated into the listening sequence to increase focus and auditory processing.

CHAPTER 2

Getting Started

The activities in this chapter are generally designed for students with greater challenges and younger students who are struggling to communicate and having difficulty with social skills and academic performance. Because they often have few readily known or socially appropriate means for communicating with others, it should not be surprising that these students may easily exhibit challenging behaviors. All activities offer multimodality communication combined with physical movement, social skills, and sensory integration to provide interactive and fulfilling learning experiences.

We strongly recommend utilizing a multimodality communication approach. Choice boards, picture exchange, visual schedules, topic boards, sign language, gestures, and integration of any device the student may already have in his or her life are examples of ways to support communication and success. After all, with the incredible growing technologies and professionally designed activities, we can hold higher expectations than was previously possible.

If visual supports are not available, they are easy to make. Just snap lots of pictures of the activities and materials. Organize the pictures into picture boards, choice boards, schedules, directions, task analysis, and books, and supplement them with gestures, signs, and facial expressions.

Body Instrument

Purpose: This activity builds body awareness and identification and vocabulary for verbs and descriptors. It increases awareness of rhythm, beats, and sounds.

Materials: Music, which can be slow or fast depending on the desired mood or outcome for the activity.

Description: The students and you sit or stand informally in a circle. You will explain how we can use our bodies as instruments. For example, we can clap with our hands or stomp with our feet (the instruction can be detailed or brief depending on the level of student). Then hold your hands up and say, "What are these? What sounds can hands make?" The students will answer or be prompted to answer, "Clap," "Snap," "Tap," and "Bang." You will then spend five to ten seconds on each action (everyone participates together). Now move on to feet and repeat, "What are these? What sounds can feet make?" The students will answer, "Stomp," "Tap," "Clomp," and "Shuffle." Again the group spends five to ten seconds making each sound. You will then turn the music on and prompt the students to clap, snap, stomp, tap, etc. to the beat.

Variations:

1. The students can focus on mouth sounds—whistle, hum, kiss, cluck, smack, etc.—to the beat.

2. The students can "Pat-a-Cake"-clap to the beat with each other.

3. Add prepositions and students can clap behind their backs, under their leg, over their head, backward, and upside-down.

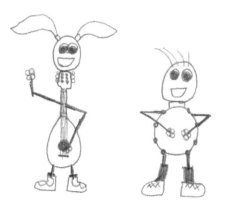

Body instruments

Co-Op Band Cooperation

Purpose: To improve strength, fitness, categorization, descriptions, expressive and receptive language, and coordination.

Materials: Exercise or co-op band. A rubber band rope can also be used. Rubber band ropes can be made by tying colorful rubber bands together.

Description: Have the students sit in a circle. Begin by passing the cord in an arm-over-arm manner. Bring the cord to a stop. When the cord is stopped, have the students name the colors. Once all the colors are named, begin passing the cord in the opposite direction. Passing can be slow, fast, medium, or a combination of all three depending on the students' ability level.

Variations:

1. When the cord is at stop, have the students use descriptive words on how the color feels or what else is that same color.

2. The students can use passing words such as "Pull like a (fill in)," "Stretch like a (fill in)," and "Pass the (fill in)."

3. As the students are sitting holding the cord, have them reach for their foot. Once they rest a hand on a part of their foot, have them name what they are touching—for example, shoes, ankle, laces, or socks.

4. Stand and hold the co-op band. You can announce, "Let's make a triangle." One person guides the group through the process of making a triangle.

Rhyming Runner

Purpose: To practice and improve auditory comprehension and discrimination, rhyming skills, general physical fitness, endurance, and bilateral coordination.

Materials: Chalk.

Description: Set up a path made of chalk on the floor for the students to follow. You can make it an oval path for easy running or make it snake around for harder running challenges. The entire path should be as long as your students can run, but a good rule of thumb is 50 meters. Every ten meters or so write out a word in chalk. The object of this game is for the runner to come to these words on the path and stop. The student will then have to say two other words that rhyme with the word on the floor. The student cannot continue running until he or she has given the answers. The play continues until the student reaches the goal.

Variations:

1. Record times to make it a competition or just for students to do their personal best.

2. You can also use antonyms or synonyms instead of rhyming words in this type of setup.

Walk Aerobics

Purpose: To work on coordination and fitness and to encourage language development. This activity strengthens the ability to follow verbal directions and follow along with a group.

Materials: Level surface such as a track or an open space.

Description: Students are to follow the directions of a peer as he or she guides them through an aerobic routine. Have the students take turns giving the following directions:

1. Walk in place for 8 counts.
2. Walk to the left for 8 counts.
3. Walk to the right for 8 counts.
5. Walk in place for 8 counts.
5. Walk forward for 8 counts.
6. Walk backward for 8 counts.
7. Walk in place for 8 counts.
8. Walk on heels for 8 counts.
9. Walk on toes for 8 counts.
10. Walk in place for 8 counts.
11. Walk heel to toe for 8 counts.
12. Walk forward crossing the legs for a count of 8.
13. Walk backward crossing the legs for a count of 8.
14. Walk in place slowly (slow motion) for a count of 8 and stop.

Variations:

1. Have the students perform the aerobics while listening to or singing a song to practice cadence.

Chair Exercises

Purpose: The purpose of this activity is to improve fitness and range of motion and to develop body awareness, cardiovascular strength, and the ability to listen and follow through with verbal instructions. It also enhances imagination and the ability to pretend.

Materials: A circle of chairs for sitting. Participants can also sit on a curb, a rock, or the floor.

Description: Have the students sit in a circle facing you. The students are to listen and follow along with the group leader. Allow a 30-second interval for each of the following exercises:

- Have the students stretch out their legs and run (a race) in the air.

- Have the group transition into a march (stomp feet up and down) in a parade.

- Transition into arm circles. Stretch out the arms to the side and circle forward. Next, circle in reverse, pretending to be a humming bird or butterfly.

- Work into the cherry picker. Raise the arms over the head and perform a grabbing motion with the hands. Students can pick nuts (walnuts or pecans) or fruit (oranges or apples).

- Shoulder shrug. Have the group raise and lower the shoulders, as if they were indicating "I don't know," for a count of 10.

- Knee touch. Raise the arms over the head and reach down and have both hands touch the knees. Perform for a count of 10. Students can do ten more knee touches alternating left hand to right knee and vice versa (crossing midline).

- From the knee touch, reach over the head and down to the feet. Perform the foot touch to a count of 10. Students can focus on crossing midline by doing ten more feet touches alternating right hand to left foot and vice versa.

- Seated jumping jack. Reach over the head and clap while tapping the feet to the floor. Complete up to a repetition of ten.

SPEECH IN ACTION

40

- Head drop. Slowly lower the head down so the chin touches the chest. Repeat to a count of 10. Students can imagine they are nodding yes or falling asleep.

- Head shake. Slowly turn the head to the left, looking over the left shoulder, and then slowly to the right, looking over the right shoulder. Students can pretend they are shaking their heads no.

- Hand close. Rest the hand on the leg with the palms up. Slowly open and close the hand to a count of 10.

Variations:

1. The chair exercises can be performed with music.

2. Students can take turns leading the exercises.

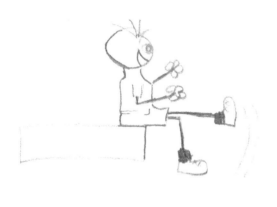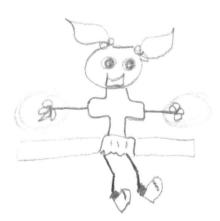

Chair exercises

Biology Analogy

Purpose: To teach analogies, body-part awareness, and identification and to practice gross motor skills.

Materials: Biology Analogy List (see below), "Table of body parts" in the Appendix.

Description: Use the set of analogies below or make up your own. Have the students get in a circle with you outside of the circle. Start off by saying the first half of the analogy and then have them take turns answering the second half of the analogy. Finally, have the students do something with that body part by saying " .... are for ...." For instance, let's say that the analogy is:

You: Gloves are to hands as socks are to ...?

Students: Feet!

You: And feet are for ...?

Students: Stomping! (or Dancing or Kicking)

Then have the students carry out the action. Have students take turns giving the answers. For this analogy call on a student to say, "Stomping," and then everyone stomps. Then call on another student who might say, "Kicking," and do that action. Continue calling on students and doing the actions until there are no more students raising their hand. Then do the next analogy on the list.

Variations:

1. If your students are good readers have them read an analogy to the class and call on other students to answer. Kids feel great pride and a sense of accomplishment when they are given the chance to lead a group, even if for just a moment.

Biology Analogy List

1. Gloves are to hands as socks are to <u>feet</u>.

2. Knit cap is to head as mittens are to <u>hands</u>.

3. Hand is to fingers as foot is to <u>toes</u>.

4. Necklace is to neck as rings are to <u>fingers</u>.

5. Sweater is to torso as pants are to <u>legs</u>.

6. Shorts are to legs as t-shirt is to <u>arms/torso</u>.

7. Shoes are to feet as helmet is to <u>head</u>.

8. Leg warmers are to legs as ear muffs are to <u>ears</u>.

9. Headband is to head as belt is to <u>waist</u>.

10. Wrapping is to presents as clothes are to <u>body</u>.

Preposition Rally

Purpose: To practice prepositions, crouching, running, standing, kneeling, crawling, giving directions, following directions, and building vocabulary.

Materials: The list of prepositions below or your own.

Description: Have the students listen to your directions and follow them safely. Your job is to give them directions verbally and they have to follow them. Use prepositions to say things like "Walk to the *front* of the room," "Crouch *under* your desk," "Get *between* two people," "Flap your arms *above* your head," or "Run to the desk in the *middle* of the room." If this exercise is done outdoors you can use outside prompts like "Stand *under* the cherry tree," "Run to the big rock *beside* the slide," or "Skip all the way to the swings and get *on* one." Have fun with this. You can make silly commands or have the students take turns making up their own preposition phrases.

Variations:

1. For beginners use prepositions that are easy to follow like *on*, *off*, *above*, *below*, *behind*, and *in front*. Have them pair up with a buddy so that if one of them doesn't know the preposition the friend can help out. Intermediate students should utilize the entire list with simple one-sentence commands. Advanced students should form complex directions like "Hop to the *outside* of the circle on one leg and then do three twirls." This helps them learn how to give directions clearly and efficiently.

Prepositions List
about, above, across, after, against, along, among, around, at, before, behind, below, beneath, beside, between, by, down, during, except, for, from, in, in front of, inside, instead of, into, like, near, of, off, on, onto, on top of, out of, outside, over, past, since, through, to, toward, under, underneath, until, up, upon, with, within, without

Raining with a Chance of Bubbles

Purpose: This activity develops hand–eye coordination, spatial relations, agility, balance, motor control, oral motor strengthening, and breath control. It promotes body-part awareness and identification.

Materials: Store-bought or homemade bubbles. For homemade bubbles you will need:

- 1 cup liquid dish soap
- 10 cups water
- 3–4 tablespoons glycerin.

The kitchen can provide a wealth of tools for making the bubble makers. Recommended items are slotted spoons, spatulas, colanders, and straws. Or use commercial plastic bubble blowers. Mix some bubble mix and pour the mix into whatever size and shape container will fit your particular bubble makers. For a large group of students a sizable container with a broad bottom is recommended.

Description: Have the students dip their bubble makers into the solution and swing or blow into their makers. The students who aren't making bubbles can run and pop bubbles, or the students can pop their own bubbles as they come off the blowers. Students can describe how their bubbles look (big, small, shiny, many, few, high, low, etc.). Use the "Table of descriptors" in the Appendix for more ideas.

Variations:

1. Have the students pop bubbles with various parts of their bodies such as head, feet, and elbows.

2. Blow the bubbles in front of a handheld battery fan and see how far the bubble can travel.

Balloon Burst

Purpose: Develops hand–eye and foot–eye coordination, reaction time, language development, verbal sequencing, oral motor strengthening, and the ability to request help.

Materials: Balloons and string.

Description: Have students blow up two balloons each and tie them around their ankles. *Do not tie onto shoelaces.* Prior to starting the activity have each student describe the task they just completed (i.e. "I blew up two balloons and tied them around my ankles"). If a student requires help with tying the balloons they should ask other students for help prior to asking you. On a designated signal students try to burst other students' balloons. After they are all popped, have the students recount what they did and how they did it (i.e. "I blew up two balloons, tied them to my ankles, and popped them like…").

Variations:

1. After the students have popped all the balloons have them name the number and colors they have popped.

2. Have students describe what the balloons sounded like when they popped.

3. Have students recall the names of others who popped their balloons and whose balloons they have popped.

Note: This activity is inappropriate for students who react negatively to loud noises.

Ma, Ma, Moo

Purpose: To practice motor planning for articulation, auditory discrimination, crossing the midline, and gross motor bilateral coordination.

Materials: Cards with targeted sounds or phonemes that the students are working on.

Description: Make as many cards per sound as there are students, minus two. For instance, if five students are playing have three "Ma" cards. Then have two "Moo" cards for the other kids. Or have three "Pa" cards and two "Pi" cards. The object is for all the students to have the same sound except for the two students who will be "it." Pick out an area clear of desks and debris. Have the students sit on the floor in a circle formation with their legs crossed. Make sure that the cards have only one sound at a time except for the two "it" cards. Pass out the cards face down and place them on the floor. Have the students take turns picking up the card in front of them and reading the sound out loud. Everyone has to pay attention because they have to figure out who are the two students who have a different sound from them. The first student who gets the "it" card becomes "it." The second student to get the "it" card has to run around the circle and hope not to get caught by the person who is "it." The round ends either when the student who is "it" catches the second "it" card or when the second student with the "it" card gets all the way around the circle once and sits back down in his or her spot. This is a Speech in Action version of Duck, Duck, Goose.

Variations:

1. Instead of sounds you can use words that have the targeted phoneme. For example, if a child is working on his or her /r/ sound, have cards with the words "red," "roll," or "rat." Be creative and find words that the kids like. "Reese's," "rocket," and "rainy" are two-syllable words for more advanced kids.

2. You can also try the phoneme in the final or middle position.

GETTING STARTED

47

Shape-Ups

Purpose: The purpose of this activity is to develop body awareness and intergroup communication and to improve coordination, endurance, listening, and following and giving directions.

Materials: None.

Description: Put the students into groups of two or three. Tell them that the purpose of this game is to make shapes using their bodies (see the illustrations below). Tell them that they can do it any way they want as long as it is safe for everybody. Explain that the shape needs to be big enough for the students to walk or crawl through. Tell them the name of the first shape. Give them time to elect a leader, talk to one another as they build the shape with their bodies, and have someone walk or crawl through. Have the students verbalize the shape name as they crawl or walk through it.

Variations:

1. Advanced: Have one student stand in front of the shapes. Call out a sequence—for example, square, circle, or triangle. The student has to travel through the shapes following the sequence that was announced.

2. Easy: Have the students just do the shapes with their hands independently of others.

SPEECH IN ACTION

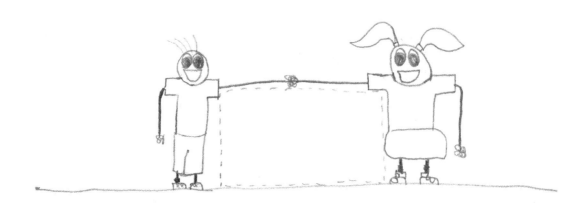

Shape-up rectangle

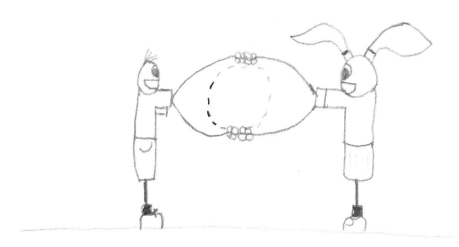

Shape-up circle

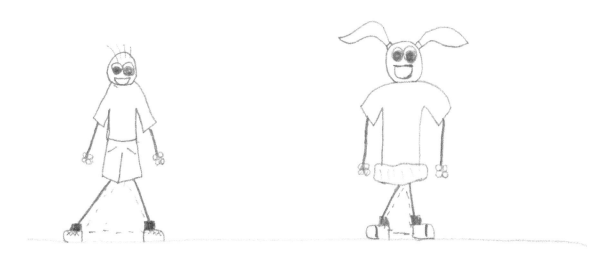

Shape-up triangles

49

Chair Soccer

Purpose: This activity will improve motor skills, body-part identification, left-to-right orientation, cooperative play, sportsmanship, visual motor integration, visual perceptual skills, bilateral coordination, kicking, and grasping.

Materials: Students can sit on the floor or in chairs set in a circle. A low-impact soccer ball or a playground ball.

Description: Once the students are in a circle, mention that they are only to use their feet, legs, or knees during the activity. Introduce the ball into the circle, and let them begin kicking it. Encourage the students to make sure all the participants receive equal time kicking the ball.

Variations:

1. Set up the chairs or sit in a circle. Have the students kick-pass from left to right, one player to another. This way the ball travels in a circle. Next reverse the direction of the ball. Have the students verbalize whose turn it is as the ball comes around. Have the group verbalize items that are round. Also have the group name objects that roll.

2. Set up the chairs or sit in a circle. Divide the group into two teams. Have enough space between the chairs or students so that the ball has the potential to slip past. The object is for one team to kick the ball outside the circle. The team that kicks the ball outside the circle is awarded the point. Encourage the teams to communicate and encourage one another and work as a unit. After the game, have the teams show good sportsmanship by shaking the hands of the other team members and saying, "Good game."

3. Have the students pass the ball to each other after saying the name of an occupation. The next student has to name another one before he or she kicks it (the "Table of occupations" in the Appendix might be useful here).

Simon Says

Purpose: This activity improves the ability to give and follow one-step directions. It increases muscle strength and range of motion and promotes good sportsmanship.

Materials: None.

Description: This is a tried and true game. Simon Says can be easily modified to fit any ability and activity level. Everyone loves Simon Says! The group can be in a circle, scattered, or lined up. There is one leader who gives directions such as "Simon says touch your toes," "Simon says spin in a circle," and "Simon says sit on the floor." Then the leader randomly gives a direction that does not include the phrase "Simon says." If anyone follows the direction they get to rest while the others continue the game. The game continues until one person is left standing. That person becomes the leader and the game begins again. You may need to lead the group several times to ensure that the rules of Simon Says are understood.

Variations:

1. Two-step directions can be given to increase difficulty as students get good at listening.

2. To really sharpen listening skills, have background music. The music can get louder and louder as students get better and better at listening.

3. The idiom "I'm all ears" can be used to describe how the students are paying attention to instructions.

Sign Language Exercise

Purpose: To improve hand–eye coordination and imagination, learn the signs A through Z, and build knowledge of descriptors, verbs, and adverbs.

Materials: Pictures of alphabet signs (see the "American Sign Language alphabet" in the Appendix).

Description: Students are to sign the alphabet letter, create a word or sentence with the letter, and perform the movement associated with the sign.

Examples:

A (sign), airplane, fly like an airplane (verbalize), and perform a movement like an airplane.

B (sign), bounce or bounce up the steps (verbalize), and mimic bouncing a ball.

C (sign), crunch (verbalize), and perform sit up.

D (sign), dangle or dangle arms to the feet (verbalize), and dangle arms to the feet.

E (sign), elastic (verbalize), and reverse arch on exercise ball.

F (sign), forward or forward march (verbalize), and forward roll on a mat.

G (sign), grab (verbalize), and grab a flag off the ground.

H (sign), hit or hit the ball (verbalize), and mimic swinging a bat.

I (sign), instant (verbalize), and create instant exercise and mimic.

J (sign), jump or jump across the river (verbalize), and perform a jump.

K (sign), kick (verbalize), and perform a kick motion.

L (sign), leap or leap like a lizard (verbalize), and perform a leap.

M (sign), move (verbalize), and mimic moving as a rabbit.

N (sign), no (verbalize), and shake head from left to right.

52

O (sign), overhead or reach arms over the head (verbalize), and perform the movement.

P (sign), push or push-up (verbalize), and perform a push-up.

Q (sign), quick (verbalize), and perform a quick movement.

R (sign), run or run like a rabbit (verbalize), and mimic running like a rabbit.

S (sign), shuffle (verbalize), and perform a shuffle to the left and to the right.

T (sign), twist (verbalize), and perform the twist dance.

U (sign), under (verbalize), and get down low on the floor to mimic crawling under a fence.

V (sign), vertical leap (verbalize), and perform a vertical leap.

W (sign), walk or walk through the woods (verbalize), and perform a brisk walk.

X (sign), xylophone (verbalize), and mimic playing the xylophone.

Y (sign), yes (verbalize), and move head up and down.

Z (sign), zip (verbalize), and mimic a zipper movement.

Variations:

1. Have students create the letter with their bodies or team up to make more difficult letters such as *H*. If there are enough students, words or their names can be spelled.

2. Students can name emotions or feelings that begin with the target letter and then act out the sentiment with facial expression and body language (use the "Table of emotions and feelings" in the Appendix for ideas).

GETTING STARTED

53

Hula-Hoop Activities

Purpose: To improve fine motor skills, visual motor integration, visual perceptual skills, bilateral coordination, imagination, left-to-right orientation, agility, grasping, and body-part awareness and identification.

Materials: Students can use a store-bought Hula-hoop.

Description: Stand with feet about one foot (30 centimeters) apart. The key is to put one foot slightly in front of the other. Place the Hula-hoop over your head and rest it against your back at your waist. Then, push the hoop around your waist and shift your weight back and forth on your feet to keep the hoop moving. Do not move your hips in circles, simply rock back and forth in a pumping motion. Try looping the Hula-hoop in both directions to find which is right for you.

Variations:

1. Hold the hoop over your body and allow the hoop to drop down without touching your body. If the hoop touches the body, name the part of the body that the hoop touches.

2. Place the hoop around your arm. Begin by rotating the arm in a forward motion. As the hoop begins to roll, it should pick up speed and roll about the arm in a circle. Challenge the students to switch the rotating hoop from left to right arm and vice versa. Count off 1-2-3, switch to the left arm, and have the group follow.

3. Drive your car. Have the group hold the hoop in front of them like a steering wheel. Now have the group imagine they are at a race track or a city road, or name a destination they would like to go to. As they begin the drive, have the group create as many race car sounds as they can imagine.

   Have the students roll the hoop to one another. Challenge the students to describe how the hoop is rolling.

4. Line up the hoops in a straight line, using no fewer than ten hoops. Have the students line up at the front of the line and step across the hoops without touching the sides. As the students travel across the line, have them say where they are going—for example, "I am stepping up to the stars" or "I am climbing a stairway to the moon." Other hoops can be arranged in side-by-side patterns or in a hopscotch pattern.

5. When the hoops are arranged on the ground, students can hop like a bunny, bounce like a ball, jump like a jackrabbit, or walk like a giant through the hoops. Students should be encouraged to make up their own similes and metaphors when traveling through the hoops.

6. Have students roll the hoops like wheels while singing "The Wheels on the Bus."

7. Last but not least, have the students hula the hoops on their hips like a hula dancer. You can prompt for trivia about Hawaii such as:

   • Where is Hawaii?

   • What language do Hawaiians speak?

   • What is a *luau*?

   • What is a *lei*?

   • What does *aloha* mean?

   • What ocean is Hawaii in?

Ball to Target

Purpose: The purpose of this activity is to improve visual motor skills and to increase knowledge of prepositions, descriptors, and spatial concepts.

Materials: Create a target. Examples are a tub, a small net, a Hula-hoop, or a cardboard box. A handheld ball, a wad of paper, a wad of aluminum foil, or a sock roll. Once the materials have been selected, arrange the distance between the target and the thrower so that chances of success are excellent.

Description: Have the students begin by throwing the ball to the target at the preferred distance. You should narrate the first round, saying, for example, "I am going to throw the ball into the round basket." After the throw you should describe the result: "It landed inside the basket" or "It landed behind the basket." Each student should get three tries at the throw. On the second round, have the students incorporate language into the activity. Examples are:

- How does it sound? Crash, bang, or boom?
- What are you throwing at?
- How does it look?
- How many landed inside the basket, outside, beside, on the left, and on the right?

Variations:

1. Have several different targets at various distances from the thrower.
2. Have the student attempt a backward throw or kick to get the ball into the receptacle.
3. Give students the opportunity to narrate for one another in the style of a golf game, soccer game, or baseball game. Provide a microphone (any cylindrical object will do) to encourage greater participation.

Tennis Ball Teasers

Purpose: The purpose of this activity is to improve visual motor skills, name identification, listening skills, visual memory, and group pragmatics, and to increase the use of verbs and adverbs.

Materials: One tennis ball or bouncing ball.

Description: Arrange the group in a circle. Decide what type of pass you are going to use. For example, you can use a bounce pass, a high bounce, a low bounce, or an underhand pass. Have the students begin by throwing the ball to one another. Start by having the students call out the name of the student they are tossing to. Next have the students use full sentences—for example, "I am going to bounce the ball to _____."

Variations:

1. Have one student perform a trick pattern with the ball—for example, dribble, toss, and catch. The student passes the ball to another, and the receiver mimics the same pattern. Have the student call out the description of the trick pattern. For example, the student can call, "toss, bounce, and spin." When each student has had a turn, have another student create a trick pattern and repeat the sequence.

Balance Time—On the Floor

Purpose: The purpose of this activity is to improve balance skills, proprioceptive abilities, body-part awareness and identification, auditory processing, and the ability to follow multistep directions.

Materials: A level surface.

Description: Students should stand in a loose circle. They will mimic each balance posture that you present to them. The goal is to get to ten seconds for each posture presented.

1. Do a deep knee bend (squat) with your arms out to the side and hold for a count of 10.

2. Stand on tiptoe and do a deep knee bend with your arms out to the side and hold for a count of 10.

3. Do a deep knee bend with your arms out to the side. From that position raise onto your toes and back down ten times.

4. Sit with your feet out in front and your knees bent at a 90-degree angle, and your arms stretched out to the sides to a count of 10.

   (a) Raise and stretch out your left leg to a count of 10. Repeat with your right leg.

   (b) Raise and stretch out both legs to a count of 10.

5. With your feet in front and your knees bent at 90 degrees, place your hands on either side of your hips and push your hips into the air to a count of 10.

   (a) Alternate raising and stretching your left and right arms and left and right legs. Rest.

   (b) Raise and stretch your right arm and left leg at the same time to a count of 10.

   (c) Raise and stretch your left arm and right leg at the same time to a count of 10.

   (d) Have the students attempt to walk (forward, backward, and sideways) in this position.

6. After a short rest, the students should move onto their hands and knees.

   (a) Alternate raising and stretching your left and right arm out in front for a count of 10.

   (b) Alternate raising and stretching your left and right legs behind and to the side for a count of 10.

   (c) Stretch your right arm out in front and your left leg to the back and around to the side slowly to a count of 10.

   (d) Stretch your left arm out in front and your right leg to the back and around to the side slowly to a count of 10.

7. Have the students get into push-up position. This position is the most challenging. Some students may choose to participate on their hands and knees.

   (a) Alternate raising and stretching your right and left arm out to a count of 10.

   (b) Alternate raising and stretching your left and right leg out to a count of 10.

   (c) This is the most challenging of all! Have the students raise their right arm and left leg to the count of 10.

   (d) Have the students raise their left arm and right leg to a count of 10.

Variations:

1. Instruct the students to identify two of their own body parts and balance with them. Switch to different parts and identify the two parts they are using to balance. Repeat the activity using three parts and four parts.

2. Begin with music and have the students move about on the floor (rolling, scooting, crab-walking, or crawling) to the song. When the music stops, the students are to freeze in that position. They must hold the position for ten seconds. After ten seconds, start the music and repeat.

3. Have the students close their eyes and do the activity. Aside from getting the giggles, they find it very challenging to keep their eyes closed.

GETTING STARTED

59

Balancing Act

Purpose: The purpose of this activity is to improve balance skills, proprioceptive abilities, body-part awareness and identification, auditory processing, creativity, and the use of descriptors.

Materials: Anything that can be balanced on the head such as beanbags, books, magazines, or backpacks.

Description: Have the students practice balancing an object on their heads while standing and walking. When they have gotten the idea of balancing something on their heads, they can take turns naming the type of "hat" they are wearing. One student may say, "I am wearing a king's crown," and then all students begin strutting like a king. Another student may announce, "I am wearing a fireman's hat," and all students act like they are putting out a fire. This goes on until all students have had a turn or two. (If the students need some inspiration for hats and the professions that wear them, see the "Table of occupations" in the Appendix.)

Variations:

1. While the students are balancing their hats on their heads, call out an action such as skip, gallop, spin, slow motion walk, or walk backward. All students should follow the direction. If hats fall off, the students can pick them up and begin again. The students can take turns calling out actions for the group to follow.

2. Musical hats is a fun game. Turn on some lively music and have the students begin dancing with their hats on. If their hat falls off, they get to sit and rest. The last person with a hat on gets to dance until it falls off.

3. Have the students experiment with different types of hats. The students can discuss which ones stay on the best and why. Why are some objects (ball) not a good choice for a hat?

"Hokey Pokey"

Purpose: This is an all-time favorite dance song. We have made some modifications to infuse language, knowledge of verbs, body-part awareness and identification, balance, coordination, left and right orientation, and listening skills.

Materials: Music for the "Hokey Pokey" is suggested but not necessary.

Description: Students stand or sit in a circle. Begin by singing (part of or all) the original "Hokey Pokey" song (see "'Hokey Pokey' lyrics" in the Appendix). When the students have the idea, begin changing the body parts to shake all around (see "Table of body parts" in the Appendix). Have the students call out names of body parts to shake all around. Change the song again by substituting various verbs for the word *shake* such as *twist, wobble, shiver, flap, pump, wave, flutter,* or *wag*. Again have the students call out a body part and a verb to use in the song. This can get really fun and silly. Last, change the verb in the phrase "turn yourself around." A student might want to use the line, "You do the Hokey Pokey and bounce yourself around." Now the "Hokey Pokey" is an entertaining and imaginative language-infused activity.

Variations:

1. Substitute names of bones for the body parts (see "Body parts and corresponding bones ('Hokey Pokey' and 'Dem Bones')" in the Appendix).

2. Students can take turns calling out the names of other participants to replace body parts. For example, students might say, "You put Alex in, you put Alex out, you put Alex in and you shake him all about." Students can also change the verb from *shake* to *roll* or *twirl*.

3. To increase auditory discrimination and knowledge of rhyming words, students can change the name of the song to any two rhyming words (e.g. "Pickle Tickle," "Oinky Doinky," or "Chunky Monkey").

Socks, Shoes, and Manners

Purpose: The purpose of this activity is twofold. First and foremost is to practice good manners. Second is to increase vocabulary, awareness of others, group pragmatics, dressing skills, and muscle flexibility.

Materials: Participants' shoes and socks, backpacks, or other personal items.

Description: Participants sit in a circle with their legs stretched out in front of them in a V shape. All participants remove their socks and shoes and place them in the middle of the circle. You will then mix them up and scatter them around making sure that the students will have to stretch to reach each item. Students take turns asking for their shoes and socks from the other students using their names and polite statements. You should model, "Excuse me Bonnie, would you please pass my sock?" The student called upon reaches the sock and passes it to the first student, saying "Here it is" or passes it to a closer student, saying "Could you pass this to Colin?" The first student then thanks the other student or students and puts the sock on. Students take turns requesting socks and shoes until they have all their items back. If students do not want to use socks and shoes, they can use other personal items such as backpacks, folders, pencils, markers, hats, coats, or sweaters.

Variations:

1. Students can practice using greetings at the beginning of the activity and salutations at the end of the activity.

2. If the students are up for a challenge, try doing this activity nonverbally using gestures, head nods, and shakes only. Facial expression can indicate a thank-you. Handshakes or waves can be used for greetings and salutations.

CHAPTER 3

Moving On

Our challenge is to help each individual use every capacity or fragment of capacity to achieve and maintain a higher level of participation and functioning. Initial sessions might be disorganized and may well appear chaotic. This *will* change—as students become familiar with the routine, participation will increase and they will look forward to each and every session. Shortly after that, you will see and hear the fruits of your labor emerge into their daily routines. Success! So, even though in the beginning you will run into challenges, stick with it. Communication combined with movement and activity is a highly effective mode of learning.

The activities in this chapter are designed to promote the language skills of describing, categorization, asking and answering questions, following multistep directions, group interactions, and turn taking, and to enhance physical awareness and abilities. All exercises are developed with goals of not only enhancing overall physical activity but also infusing, encouraging, and teaching important communication skills.

While it is true that some individuals with disabilities may be resistant to exercise, we hope that participants will pursue healthy, active lifestyles; have fun; and stave off problems later in life. Obesity, coronary artery disease, and diabetes may be prevented with regular activity. Again, start slow and make it fun, and they will participate willingly.

Category Catch

Purpose: To develop catching, throwing, categorization, and sequencing skills.

Materials: Ball. (See Variations below if you don't have a ball.)

Description: Have the students arrange themselves in a circle or face each other if there are only two people. Give them each a baseball glove if you want to work with those. If you will be using a glove use a small, soft ball, and if you will not be using the glove then use a large ball. Have one of the students pick a category that he or she likes then start out by saying one of the items in the category and then throw the ball to another student. For example, student A picks "cartoons" as the category and then says "Sponge Bob" as he or she throws the ball to student B. Student B then says "Pokémon" and throws the ball to the next student. This keeps going on until somebody says an item that has already been said or the ball has gone around the circle for a long time.

Variations:

1. If you don't have a ball you can get a bunch of newspaper pages and wad them up into the shape of a ball. You can keep it together by adding pieces of tape as needed.

2. Another variation of this game is to use a sequential action and have each student tell you one of the steps. Student A picks the category "making a pizza." Then student B says the first action: "Get the dough." Student C says, "Put tomato sauce on the dough." Student D says, "Add cheese on top," and the sequence continues until the action has been completed.

Look at Me!

Purpose: Promotes eye contact, paying attention, crossing midline, hand–eye coordination, and hand speed. This game focuses the student's attention to the eyes. It teaches how to look at the eyes of people in order to get information. It is a great game for students who have a hard time looking at people—they can play a fun game and learn to make more eye contact at the same time.

Materials: None.

Directions: This game was adapted from a children's game that is popular in my school. It is very much like the game "hot hands." The game starts by placing yourself in front of a student. Place your hands out with the palms facing up. The student places his or her hands directly above your hands, facing down, but does not touch them. The object of the game is to try to touch the student's hands by flipping one of your hands and lightly touching the top of the student's hand. The student has to retract his or her hands quickly in order to avoid them being touched. You will try to make it easier for the student by giving him or her clues with your eyes. When you look down at your right hand the student will have to remove the hand that is placed above this hand in order to prevent it getting touched. If the student's hand is touched the teacher gets a point. If the student's hand is removed before it can be touched the student gets the point.

Variations:

1. For students who need instant rewards you might want to think about using preferred items or edibles. Instead of keeping points have Gummi Bears, cheese crackers, raisins, little wind-up toys, tops, or any other consumables at hand to give to the student after each point he or she makes. A consumable is a reward that will get used up or eaten in a few seconds. If you do not use consumables you might find yourself in a tug-of-war with the student for their favorite toy once it's time to resume play.

Follow That Cat-egory

Purpose: To develop categorization skills, balance, speed, and agility through a fun game.

Materials: Cards with pictures from two categories and chalk.

Description: Carefully trace a straight line on the floor about five feet (one and a half meters) long. Draw four more lines in different shapes, for example zigzag lines, S-shaped lines, wiggly lines, diagonal lines or looped lines, each parallel to the first. Put one picture at the end of each line. The teacher can pick two students; each one should be assigned a category such as "toys" or "food." Have the students walk the line and then pick up the first picture. Then have the student walk the line back, but this time have him or her do it backward to the beginning again. Once finished the student has to decide what category the picture belongs to and then hand the picture to the appropriate student. Have the other students run through the lines as quickly as they can while still staying within the boundaries. After the five pictures are picked up, add another five and then have them go through it again.

Variations:

1. Magazines are great substitutes for pictures. Pages can be easily ripped out and used instead of more formal cards or pictures.

2. Speed race—have the students race through the lines to see who wins.

3. Personal best—time the students to see how fast they get through the course.

4. Noncompetitive—students try their best one at a time.

Hopscotch

Purpose: To strengthen jumping and balancing abilities, increase articulation of specific phonemes, and practice categorization and oral motor exercises.

Materials: Open space, chalk, and index cards.

Description: Draw a hopscotch form on the floor. The next step can be to either draw on the inside of each square or to place an index card inside each hopscotch box (see the illustration below).

- Oral motor activity: Put pictures of different mouth positions and tongue positions on index cards and scatter a few throughout the hopscotch form. As the student jumps through the form have him or her mimic the mouth position. You can also draw the positions if you have chalk.

- Articulation activity: Draw a letter or a sound blend that the student is working on in each of the squares (/r/ or /s/). As the student jumps have him or her shout the sound or blend out loud.

- Categorization activity: Write categories on index cards and place the stack on the floor next to the hopscotch form. Before the students begin their run through the form have them pick out a card and read it out loud. Then the child has to say items belonging to that category as he or she jumps through.

Variations:

1. If you don't have index cards you could use your own face to show examples of what the mouth positions should look like. For instance, you could open your mouth wide or stick out your tongue. For the categories you could approach the hopscotch form with the students and say each category (e.g. "cartoon characters," "food," "emotions," etc.).

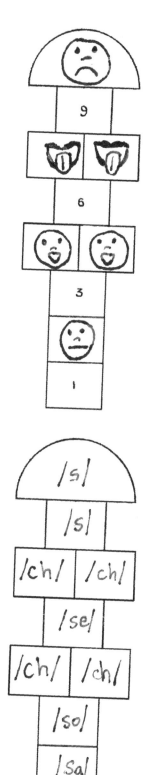

Hopscotch forms

67

Musical Paper Plates

Purpose: To develop hand–eye coordination, endurance, mobility, spatial awareness, listening skills, language, and grammar.

Materials: Paper plates or cardboard pizza rings. Have the plate or ring labelled with a color (blue) and a verb (*hop, skip, gallop, strut, swagger,* or *crab-walk*) and lively music.

Description: Each student is assigned a colored plate. Arrange the plates on the floor in a large circle. Have the students stand on a plate. Begin the music. The students are to listen to the music and walk in a circle as the music plays. When the music stops ask, "What do you have?" The students say the color and verb they are standing on in a sentence (e.g. "I have a blue *skip*"). The music starts again and all students move according to the verb. Once again the music stops and you begin the sequence again.

Variations:

1. After each round, remove one plate. Play resumes similar to musical chairs. When the music stops, the students are to leap onto the plates. The student who does not land on a plate moves to the middle of the circle and sits quietly while the others finish. The game continues until one student is left.

2. Plates can have names of categories on them. When the music stops each student gets to name three items from his or her category.

Clean Your Room

Purpose: To increase flexibility, have fun, and encourage teamwork. To build group pragmatics, endurance, and the use of descriptors.

Materials: Wads of paper, aluminum foil, or rolled socks.

Description: This activity works best with groups of six or more. Students are given one to three sheets of newspaper or aluminum foil to crumple into a ball. The students are divided into two teams. Mark a centerline with chalk, tape, cones, or a net. On the signal, the students are to throw the paper or foil to the opposing team. On the second signal, the players stop and the team with the least amount of paper is the winner. The students are to count the wads of paper or foil and describe how the paper is flying (e.g. "like a hailstorm") and what the floor looks like after the play is over. Use the "Table of descriptors" in the Appendix for ideas.

Variations:

1. Students can kick, toss, or bat the paper or foil over the midline with their hands.

2. Students must not face one another and should have their backs to the midline.

3. Students can team up. One student can pitch and the other can bat, kick, swat, or bump the paper or foil over the midline.

Tongue Twister

Purpose: To work on hand–eye coordination, listening skills, articulation, and expressive language development.

Materials: Any quiet open area.

Description: Have the students recite the tongue twisters below. Next, using different parts of their body, have them clap out the rhythm of the tongue twisters. Rhythm instruments can also be used.

Tongue twisters:

- Which witch wished first?
- For fine fresh fish, phone Phil.
- Weary railroad works.
- He who laughs last laughs late.
- Theopholous the thistle sifter.
- A fish sauce shop.
- Seven crisp snacks.
- Bob's blue blobs.
- Slick silk socks.
- Zack's knapsack strap.

Variations:

1. Have the students recite the tongue twisters as they are passing a ball around.

2. Have each student assigned to a tongue twister. When a student comes into contact with the ball he or she recites the twister before passing the ball to another student.

3. Have each student recite a word as her or she comes into contact with the ball.

Catching Scoops

Purpose: To improve reaction time, one-to-one correspondence, spatial awareness, and visual motor skills.

Materials: Half-gallon empty bleach bottles, scissors, string, and a lightweight plastic ball. Using scissors cut off the bottom of the bleach bottle. Now cut a U-shape on the same side as the handle. Punch a hole in the wall of the bottle about half an inch (one centimeter) from the outer edge. Measure and cut a length of string of about 24 inches (60 centimeters). Tie one end through the punched hole in the bottle and the other end to a lightweight plastic ball. The string should be easy to tie and untie from the plastic scoop and ball.

Description: Participants are to team up in groups of two to ten students. Each participant should have a scoop. Group size can range from two to ten persons. Using the ball, stand about six feet (two meters) apart. Prior to tossing the ball, the students should call out the name of their partner and obtain eye contact. Begin tossing and catching the ball with the scoops. See how many times the ball can be caught without dropping it.

Variations:

1. Participants can tie their string and ball onto the scoop for individual practice with String Ball Scoop. Hold the scoop so that the ball is nearly touching the ground. Swing the arm in an upward motion. Watch the ball as it swings up. Once the ball is up in the air, try to catch it with your scoop. Encourage students to name things that can be caught or scooped (e.g. baseball, fly, football, butterfly, etc.).

2. Students can count catches for each other and then report, "Tomas caught seven balls in a row."

MOVING ON

71

Dancing Ribbons

Purpose: To improve coordination, body awareness, endurance, and receptive and expressive language, and to promote leadership and imagination.

Materials: Dancing ribbons; scarves or pom-poms.

Description: Each student is given a dancing ribbon. Begin the activity by having the students experiment with the various shapes the ribbon can make. Examples are free form, circles, back and forth, overhead, up and down, and corkscrew. Next name and model the forms: twirl, side to side, overhead, up and down, and circle. Have the students describe how the ribbon moves. Each student takes a turn being the leader by choosing what form to move the ribbon in and what it looks like. The group joins along.

Variations:

1. The ribbons are an ideal activity for following the music. Pick songs that have clear lyrics—for example, "Twist and Shout" by The Beatles or "Cupid Shuffle."

2. Students can collaborate to make a routine and give a performance.

3. Dance steps can be added by you or the students as appropriate.

Dance, Dance, Dance

Purpose: To improve muscle strength, endurance, coordination, listening skills, and awareness of others. To stimulate imagination and interpretation of dance styles and moves.

Materials: Music!

Description: The students and you assemble in an informal circle. Name several dances and have the students practice them. Examples of dances include swim, dive, mashed potatoes, worm, twist, churn the butter, sprinkler, robot, break dance, monkey, jitterbug, Charleston, running man, and jerk. Then start the music and call out a dance name. Students are encouraged to observe others and help others who do not know the dance well. After about a minute, call out the name of a different dance and have all participants engage in that dance. The students will usually participate until the end of the period or until exhausted.

Variations:

1. Use line dances such as the Macarena or electric slide.

2. Partner up for square dancing, the bump, or a waltz.

3. Make a competition: Call out a dance and begin the music. All participants dance. When the music stops, all participants freeze. The last person to freeze gets to sit and rest until the competition is over.

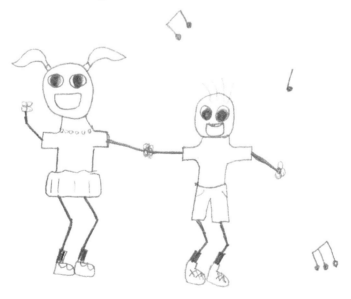

Dance, Dance, Dance

Mr. Wolf, What Time Is It?

Purpose: To work on coordination, endurance, listening skills, one-to-one correspondence, concept of time, teamwork, and language development.

Materials: Any wide-open area.

Description: This is a tag variation. One person is "it" or the wolf. The group lines up in the safety zone. The safety zone can be in front of a wall or in a set of rings. As a group the students ask the wolf, "Mr. Wolf, what time is it?" The wolf says, "Two o'clock", and the students take two steps out of the safety zone. Again the students ask, "Mr. Wolf, what time is it?" The wolf replies, "Six o'clock", and the students take six steps forward. Now when the students ask Mr. Wolf what time it is, if the wolf says midnight the students have to run back to the safety zone. If the students get tagged, they automatically become part of the wolf's team. The game continues until all of the students have been tagged.

Variations:

1. Game can be played in slow or fast motion.

2. Game can be played like freeze tag. When students are tagged, they freeze. If they are retagged by a safe student, they can move again. The last person tagged gets to be the wolf.

Mystery Moves

Purpose: To increase awareness of synonyms and antonyms while acting out a physical action of the words.

Materials: Index cards with synonyms (set 1) and antonyms (set 2) printed on them with pictures. See the synonyms and antonyms lists in the Appendix for more ideas.

Description: Pass out one card with pictures to each student from the synonyms set. When you have handed them all out tell the students to look at their picture and pantomime what they see. Have them act out the synonym as long as necessary until they find someone doing the same thing. Have the students find their synonym pair and move aside to the wall. Once everyone has paired up have them show what their synonym was to the class by taking turns. Start over but this time use the antonyms card set.

Synonyms	Antonyms
jumping/bouncing	stand/sit
walking/strolling	hands up/hands down
wiggling/shaking	push/pull
sit-ups/crunches	in/out
turning/twirling	still/moving
shouting/yelling	signaling to come/leave
skip/hop	excited/bored

Variations:

1. Have the students ask for their preferred partner using full sentences and appropriate grammar. Then give them a set of synonyms that they must act out in front of the class. The entire class has to guess what the pair is acting out. Once the class has guessed the action correctly have a different pair come up. Do this with the antonyms too.

Role-Playing Holiday Manners

Purpose: To develop social pragmatics, problem solving, role-playing, acting out words with movement, and using hands and body to gesture.

Materials: None.

Description: Have the students sit at their desks except for two students who will be chosen to do the role-playing. Give them one of the scenarios and ask them to use their bodies and their words to convey the message they want to get across. Tell them to act as polite as they can but to also be true to themselves. In this activity we are trying to teach them alternative ways to act in a social situation during the holidays. Try to teach them appropriate manners. Make sure to emphasize that body language also *tells* people how we feel and that if they have a scowl on their face as they greet their relatives then the scowl will say more than their words. Switch off pairs of students until everyone has had a turn.

Role-playing scenarios:

- Your family will need *your* room for a guest spending Christmas night.

- Your aunt pinches your cheeks when she greets you and you want to tell her to stop. How can we tell her without hurting her feelings? When is it okay?

- Guests bring food that seems gross to you and then ask how you liked their dish.

- You have to wear an uncomfortable suit or dress and you don't want to.

- Your parents ask you to be the greeter and you have to let everyone in. How do we greet family members? How do we greet strangers? Friends?

- Your parents ask you to help clean the house after the party. How can you bargain with them to get the chores you would prefer to do?

- You are saying grace at dinner (a thank you for the food and company). Give them ideas of what to say and have them practice these so they feel comfortable with it.

76

Variations:

1. With beginners, practice greetings, opening the door, taking coats as they talk, saying goodbye appropriately, looking people in the eyes, and shaking hands. Intermediate and advanced students should concentrate on appropriate responses to the social situations. When can we protest? Why do we have to fake liking food sometimes? Why do we have to do things we don't like? Explore these questions with your students at the end.

Rope Exercises

Purpose: The purpose of this activity is to improve coordination, range of motion, and visual perception, and to develop body awareness, imagination, group participation, and pragmatics. The activity also creates an awareness of metaphors and similes.

Materials: Use a three-foot-long rope for the exercises. Follow each picture on the exercise sheet (see page 79) and model it for the students.

Description: Have the students hold the rope. Have the group leader model the exercises for the students. Perform each movement for a count of 5. As the students perform each movement have them create a word or words to describe the movement. For example, side to side can be described as a "rock," twisting can be like a "top," and shaking can be like "a leaf on a tree."

Variations:

1. Students can team up using both ropes or just one to create unique movements.

2. Students can mirror each other's movements.

3. Students can make a rope chain by holding on to the ends of the rope, alternating rope with student. The leader then calls out an action. The students move as a group performing that action and working to keep the chain intact.

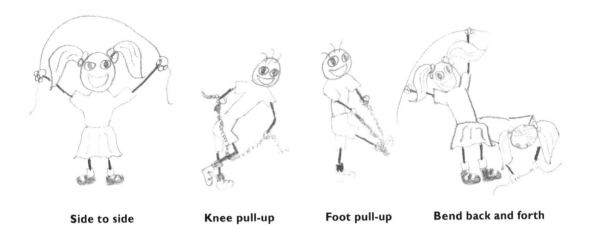

Side to side   **Knee pull-up**   **Foot pull-up**   **Bend back and forth**

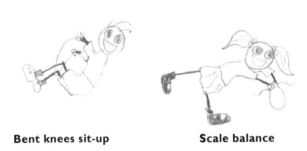

Bent knees sit-up   **Scale balance**

Rope exercises

Chalk Course

Purpose: The purpose of this activity is to improve mobility and range of motion, and to develop body awareness, community awareness, cardiovascular strength, and group pragmatic skills. This activity is lots of fun!

Materials: Colored chalk, track, and a city block or playground.

Description: Using the colored chalk, have each student draw an image of a person doing a particular exercise. Examples include someone performing jumping jacks, toe touches, or waist turns. Then gather the students and lead them to a starting mark. Explain to the group as they walk to keep their eye out for drawings. When they find a drawing they will perform the illustrated activity ten times. When you encounter the drawing have the student verbalize the action in the illustration. When the exercise is completed have each student move to the next picture.

Variations:

1. When moving between the pictures, have one of the students say to the group, "Hop to the next picture."

2. When students find a picture, they can balance on their left foot.

3. As the students are walking, have them identify objects that are colored blue. Have the students name the cars as they walk. Have the students identify sounds they hear in the community.

4. Turn the walk into a type of scavenger hunt where the students collect and identify items they have gathered.

Arctic Artic

Purpose: To practice articulation, throwing, aiming, and crumpling.

Materials: Pieces of scratch paper, a container, and pencils.

Description: Have the students write words related to their articulation goals on pieces of paper and then have them crumple up the paper into "snowballs." Set up a container, shoes, a wastebasket, or a box a few feet away from the students. Tell the students that they can go on your mark and throw the snowballs into the receptacle. Once everyone has thrown all their snowballs, take the canister and read aloud the articulation prompt (the word) for the students to repeat. If there are more snowballs on the ground have them read the ones that missed, but if there are more inside the canister then read those. It's all about having them do as much articulation as possible while still having a blast.

Variations:

1. If your students are able to tolerate the fun that comes with a snowball fight give everyone his or her own receptacle and then have them throw the balls at each other's containers for added friendly competition.

2. This activity can be used for many language goals such as descriptions, categorization, conversation starters, and synonyms and antonyms (see the lists and tables in the Appendix for ideas).

3. If the students are really good at making baskets, place a fan in the path of the snowball to increase difficulty and build skill.

Scavenger Hunt in the Park

Purpose: To develop interpersonal communication, cooperative language, walking, crouching, stretching, and following multistep directions.

Materials: None necessary, but an optional quick list of actions for the hunt is recommended to make it fun and to see who finishes first.

Directions: Take your students to a park and divide them into pairs. If you decide not to use a list then have the students in each pair take turns calling out the orders and following them. For instance the first student can say, "Find a tree and jump under it two times." Then the second student has to follow the first student's order. Next it is the first student's turn to receive the order and play out the action requested by the second student. If you decide to make a quick scavenger hunt list then place a few orders for the students to follow and have them do it simultaneously. The first to check off everything on his or her list wins. A scavenger hunt list would look like this:

- ☐ Find a tree and jump under it twice.
- ☐ Scream "Hooray" as you go down the slide.
- ☐ Twirl around while you sing "Twinkle Twinkle Little Star."
- ☐ Bounce up and down six times while saying "Boing, boing."
- ☐ Swing ten times on the swings and count out loud.

Variations:

1. If your student cannot read you can create your own pictures or print out some pictures of actions from the Internet. For a challenge try having your students mime the directions to a partner who has to do the action.

Safari Search

Purpose: To teach prepositions, gross motor movement, articulation, speaking in full sentences, listening to and following directions, walking, skipping, and other actions as directed.

Materials: Ten pictures of wild animals, a cargo vest (optional), and a safari hat (optional).

Directions: Print out about ten pictures of wild animals from the Internet and tape on various locations around your classroom. Choose one student to be the tour guide and put the safari hat on him or her. Now choose a student to be the tourist and have the tourist put on the cargo vest. The tourist asks the guide to "guide" him or her to one of the animals. The guide gets to direct the tourist with verbal directions through the classroom maze of tables, desks, bookcases, etc. to the location where the chosen animal is taped on the wall. The guide can say things like, "Go over the Legos, walk under the flag, and turn to the right." The orders are followed until the student gets in front of the animal picture. Once the tourist arrives at the destination the guide says, "Oh no, our tourist got eaten by the (chosen animal). We need another tourist!" Then the play resumes with a new student tourist. Once the guide has gotten three tourists eaten the guide is "fired" and a new guide must be chosen.

Variations:

1. You can make binoculars out of paper rolls in art class to use for this activity. You can also get an old camera and have the students take pictures of their animals. For articulation practice use animals that begin with the desired sound—for instance, leopard, lion, lizard, and locust would be chosen for the /l/ sound.

MOVING ON

83

Milk Carton Activities

Purpose: To improve mobility, fitness, hand–eye coordination, endurance, cardiovascular strength, cooperative learning, antonyms, synonyms, and giving directions, and to practice using encouragements.

Materials: Waxed half-gallon milk cartons, tennis balls or beanbags, and duct tape. Rinse out the milk cartons. Allow to dry and then cut along the upper folds of the carton. There should be four cuts. Fold down the top carton and duct tape it down. One option is to stuff the cartons with newspaper. This will give the cartons more outer durability. Once assembled you are ready to go.

Description:

- Two Two-Person Relay: Form two lines of equal numbers. For each line two students will begin the relay. The starter will place and balance a carton between the two students' shoulders. Once everyone is in place, the relay can begin. The two players will walk briskly while holding the carton between their shoulders. They have to communicate effectively in order for the carton to stay in place while they walk fast. They walk to the target and loop around the end. Once they reach the end, they hand off the carton to the next pair. If the carton is dropped before the finish, the pair needs to walk back to the beginning and start over. Encourage the players waiting to shout out encouragements or directions to their teammates.

- Carton Bowling: Set up the activity by building a pyramid of cartons. Six works best with three on the bottom, two in the middle, and one on the top. Ask the student to give you an antonym or a synonym for a word you give him or her from your list. Have the student stand at least six feet (two meters) away from the cartons. Have the student throw a tennis ball toward the cartons to see how many he or she can knock down. Beanbags can be used in place of tennis balls.

Sponge Target

Purpose: To improve fine motor skills, visual motor integration, visual perceptual skills, throwing, and grasping. This activity also develops body-part awareness and identification and increases the ability to display and interpret emotions.

Materials: A chalkboard or a wall, colored chalk, two-by-three-inch (five-by-eight-centimeter) sponges, and a bowl with water. Mount a chalkboard on an easel on the wall, or just use the wall. Cut the sponges in two-by-three-inch shapes. Use about six to ten sponges. Place the sponges in the bowl with water.

You may wish to set up a throwing zone; you can arrange this by placing cones or by drawing a ring with the chalk for the students to stand in.

Description: Begin the activity by showing the students pictures of emotional faces. Next the class is going to draw an emotional face on the chalkboard or wall. Have each student begin by drawing a line or two on the chalkboard. Have each student contribute some type of detail to the face. Ask the students what the emotion is. Name the parts of the face such as eyes, nose, or ear. Describe the hair: bald, thick, or curly. When the face is complete, the sponge-throw can begin.

- Face Splat: Have the students stand about six to eight feet (two to two and a half meters) away from the target. Have the students take a sponge and throw it at the target. When the moist sponge hits the target it will leave a wet mark on it. Repeat until each student has had a throw.

- Bull's-Eye: Draw a bull's-eye-style target with numbers to record scores. Another target drawing can be of a baseball diamond.

Variations:

1. Use squirters or sprayers instead of sponges.

2. Make sponge splats on a blank chalkboard or wall and have students use chalk to create pictures from the splats.

Memory Run

Purpose: To work on hand–eye coordination, endurance, listening skills, nouns, verbs, encouragement, and short-term memory skills.

Materials: Use items in the immediate environment.

Description: Students are to listen to the instruction of the running pattern and then follow the pattern.

- Have the students line up at the starting point, and then instruct them to run to the table, touch the table, and run back.

- From the starting point the students run with the baton toward an object—for example, the trash can—tap it three times on the object, and skip back to the starting point.

- From the starting point have the students run to the tree, touch the tree, run to a table, circle the table, jump up three times, and then run back to the finish.

- From the starting point students will run for 20 steps, twirl three times, skip for six, and gallop to the starting point.

- Have the students create their own running pattern. The students are to observe the movements, then remember them and replicate the movement run.

Variations:

1. Give instructions in writing or picture sequences.

2. Give either written or verbal instructions and have the students complete tasks in reverse.

Foot Croquet

Purpose: The purpose of this activity is to improve endurance, visual motor skills, knowledge of prepositions, verbs, and descriptors, and group pragmatics.

Materials: For this activity you will need one kickball and markers (stakes, cups, or cones). Arrange the markers side by side, wide enough for the ball to pass through. A minimum of four is suggested. Arrange a start and finish for the course. Course arrangements can be of shapes, letters, or random.

Description: Have the student begin by foot dribbling to the first target. When the student is in range of the target, he or she must kick the ball between the markers. Students are encouraged to state where and how the ball went (e.g. "Quickly through the cones" or "Bouncing over the stakes"). They are also encouraged to state where the ball landed ("My ball landed behind the cone" or "My ball is between the fence and the stake"). Then they move on to the next target.

Variations:

1. During the setup of the markers, have the students collaborate and agree on the kicking trail pattern.

2. Have the students pick a list of animals with wide mouths. A hippo is one example. As the students dribble the ball to the marker, name the animal that they are kicking the ball into. As their language develops, they can move on to other statements such as "Catch it Mr. Alligator" or "Eat it Mr. Hippo."

3. Have students roll or toss the ball bocce-style instead of kicking it.

Balance Time

Purpose: The purpose of this activity is to improve balance skills, proprioceptive abilities, body-part awareness and identification, auditory processing, and the ability to follow multistep directions.

Materials: A level surface.

Description: In front of a group of students, ask the students to mimic each balance posture presented to them. The goal is to get to ten seconds for each posture presented.

- Stand with feet together and arms out to the sides.
- Stand with feet together and hands on hips.
- With arms out and feet apart squat down to a count of 10.
- Place feet apart, place arms on hips, and squat down to a count of 10.
- Stand on toes with arms out to the sides.
- Stand on toes with hands on hips.
- Stand on heels with arms out to the sides.
- Stand on heels with hands on hips.
- Stand with one foot in front of the other. The heel and toe should be touching. Position arms out to the sides and then to the hips. Repeat the exercise with the other foot in front.
- Stand on one foot with arms out to the sides. Then repeat with the other foot. Next try with hands on hips.

Variations:

1. Instruct the students to identify two of their own body parts (using the "Table of body parts" in the Appendix if necessary) and balance with them. Switch to different parts and identify the two parts they are using to balance. Repeat the activity using three parts and four parts.

2. Begin with music and have the students move about to the song (rolling, dancing, scooting, crab-walking or crawling). When the music stops, the students are to freeze in that position. They must hold the position for ten seconds. After ten seconds, start the music and repeat. Students do not necessarily have to be on the floor.

3. Have students close their eyes and do the activity. Aside from getting the giggles, they find it very challenging to keep their eyes closed.

Water Play

Purpose: To develop spatial relations and muscle strength and to improve overall physical fitness. Water Play strengthens language acquisition for synonyms, antonyms, verbs, adjectives, and adverbs. This is a highly motivational activity and lots of fun.

Materials: Any water source: sprinkler, inflatable pool, hose, squirters, water balloons, spray bottles, or city pool. Students will need clothes that they can get wet and a towel.

Description: After the students have changed into clothes that can get wet, have them sit in a group while you talk about the benefits of water. We need water to live (our bodies are 70 percent water) and we use water to clean and make our plants grow, but the best part of water is playing in it! After the students have settled back down, introduce the water source (pool squirters, hose, etc.). The students can then inflate the pool, hook up the hose, or fill the squirters or balloons. You can use this time to introduce the language concepts of *wet* and *dry, full* and *empty*. Once play begins, verbs, adverbs, and adjectives can be used to describe various activities surrounding water play. The students should be allowed free play time to explore the water themselves. All students should participate in a quiet time of lying in the sun on their towels and drying off. Language concepts of *dry, warm, relaxing,* and *resting* should be explored (deep breathing is a good cool-down for this activity). After the Water Play activity, all students will participate in cleanup and storing the water toys for another day. Dry clothes should be put back on and wet clothes should be hung in the sun to dry.

Variations:

1. A trip to the city pool can be planned by the students. City pool rules and manners should be reviewed and practiced prior to visiting the pool.

What's Your Favorite Recipe?

Purpose: This is a good stretching activity for all muscles. It promotes creativity, imagination, descriptive abilities, and verbal sequencing.

Materials: No materials required, just imagination. Background music is always nice if available.

Description: All participants should sit in a large circle with legs stretched out in front of them in a V shape. Begin by asking, "What recipe shall we make today?" The first student who raises his or her hand and answers (e.g. "Let's make cookies today") gets their recipe made. Then ask, "What do we need to make cookies?" Students usually answer, "We need flour." Model reaching behind yourself to pick up a scoop of flour and put it into the bowl (the middle of the circle). All students do the same. "What else do we need?" you ask. The students will call out an ingredient, reach behind themselves, get the ingredient, and put it into the bowl. After all the ingredients are put into the bowl, students are to stir until mixed thoroughly. Last they throw it into the oven by reaching to the middle of the circle and throwing their arms into the air. Finally after the cookies have baked, it is time to eat them: "Yummy, yummy! Now we need some milk. Let's milk the cow" (students make the milking motion with their hands).

Variations:

1. This activity has worked well with tossed salad, pizza, smoothies (the blender is particularly fun), root beer floats, and hamburgers. Let students use their imaginations.

CHAPTER 4

Feelings and Figurative Language

In this chapter we are tackling the obscure concepts of feelings and figurative language.

Let's start with feelings. Feelings may be a difficult thing for some individuals with disabilities to comprehend and more tricky to express. Facial expressions are a mystery.

Being able to express thoughts of love, friendship, pain, frustration, and empathy are all essential to emotional happiness. Not having the ability to read feelings of anger may put an individual in a dangerous situation. Every individual will benefit from participating in the activities that focus on feelings.

Remember, use visual supports! The use of visual supports will benefit all participants. Don't forget, a visual support can be *you*. Your facial expressions and gestures can supplement pictures and words. Pictures do not have to be fancy. They can be hand-drawn, cut from a magazine, drawn on a board, or pictures of the students themselves and friends. Pictures do not need to come from expensive programs to be effective. Using visuals is an extremely effective way to enhance comprehension of any lesson.

The ability to express and understand feelings can be greatly improved. Practice, practice, and practice. As a result of frequent practice and role-play an individual's ability to understand, show emotions, and read body language becomes natural rather than intellectual. Even so, be prepared to accept limitations as some individuals may struggle a lifetime to master the complex world of emotions.

Parents of individuals with autism may believe the *myth* that their children cannot feel or express love and empathy. The fact is that most people with autism are extremely capable of feeling and expressing love, though in idiosyncratic ways. Some believe that individuals on the spectrum are far more empathetic than the average person; however, they express their empathy in unusual ways. It is our challenge to bridge the communication gap that prevents the clear understanding of one another's feelings and intentions.

Let's move on to figurative language. The English language is rich because of the magnitude of vocabulary and abundant use of figurative language. Some individuals with autism learn language intellectually. Because of this they are highly literal in how they use and understand language. Small talk is all but impossible, and metaphors and idioms are more akin to lies. They lack appreciation for body language and nonverbal communication and thus cannot pick up on hints and clues that people drop. Starting or participating in a conversation is awkward without a good understanding of figurative language.

Figurative language has to be taught and explained in detail. Once again repetition and visual cues are imperative. Practice, practice, practice, and have fun.

Action Food

Purpose: To improve balance, agility, speed, muscle strength, and endurance; to increase concept and vocabulary development for action words, similes, and descriptors; and to promote imagination and a good time.

Materials: Fun or lively music.

Description: Stand at the front of the class and announce, "Today we are going to act like food." Then demonstrate a few food similes (e.g. "Pop like popcorn," "Twist like a pretzel," or "Boil like water"). When you say, "Pop like popcorn," do a few deep knee bends and pop up after each one. You can bend at the waist and wrap arms around legs for "Twist like a pretzel," and have your whole body in motion for "Boil like water." The students will interpret the action word similes to their own abilities.

- Sizzle like bacon.
- Freeze like ice cream.
- Melt like butter.
- Pop up like toast.
- Stick like candy.
- Twist like licorice.
- Snap like a pea.
- Jiggle like jelly.
- Stretch like taffy.
- Shake like a milkshake.
- Run like water.
- Peel like a banana.

Variations:

1. You can say only the first part of the simile (e.g. "Sizzle like a _____"), and the students can fill in the food that fits the action. This variation is usually very interesting and amusing.

2. Students can make their own action food similes and share.

3. Use mirrors if available or have students mirror each other's actions.

Slang Dunk

Purpose: To develop figurative language, slang, idioms, definitions, throwing, aiming, and ball control through a fun game.

Materials: Ball and basketball hoop (optional)—see Variations below.

Description: Give the students a slang term from the list provided, and then have them tell you what it means. If they get the correct, answer they can slam-dunk the ball into the basketball hoop. But if they don't know the answer they can give you an educated guess, and then, if they are correct, they have the opportunity to shoot the ball from the free-throw line. The trick here is that most students want to slam-dunk, so they will work hard to try to learn the terms you give them.

- Slang: Use the "Slang Terms" list in the Appendix for some suggestions.

- Definitions: Grab a list of words from their spelling assignments or English homework and have the students define them.

- Idioms: Use the "Idioms List" in the Appendix for some suggestions.

Variations:

1. If you don't have a basketball and a basketball hoop, use a ball made out of crumpled-up newspapers held together with tape. Then you can use an old box or a wastebasket to try to throw the ball into.

Emotional Movement

Purpose: Students will have practice interpreting and displaying emotions while following directions and learning verbs. They will increase body awareness and range of motion.

Materials: "Table of emotions and feelings" in the Appendix, with quiet background music such as classical.

Description: The students stand in a large circle at least an arm's length apart. You will review and have the class display several emotions (facial and body). At this time, the students may discuss causes of the particular emotion. Begin the routine by giving a direction such as, "Everyone move happily to the right." Movement can be: left, right, forward, backward, skipping, galloping, stiffly, rubbery, etc. Then you or a student can choose another emotion and movement (e.g. "Everyone move angrily to the left").

Variations:

1. The activity can be made more difficult by adding extra movement (e.g. "Take five steps to the left and do jumping jacks").

2. Try slow movements with eyes closed or one eye closed.

I'm a Mime

Purpose: To develop body awareness and awareness of others, follow nonverbal directions, practice body language, and improve balance and agility.

Materials: None needed.

Description: You are the only person to talk in this activity. Explain that mimes exaggerate the actions of others; however, they do not make a sound. Then state and begin an action and instruct the students to exaggerate the action. Each action can be performed for 30 seconds to two minutes. Encourage students to watch with their eyes, listen with their ears, and let their mouth rest.

Say and perform the following actions:

- Take a stroll…Trip on a rock.
- Freeze and melt.
- Hopscotch.
- Throw a football.
- Ballet dance.
- Jump rope…Backward… Faster…Slow motion.
- Climb a mountain.

- Walk in water…Over hot coals. …On ice (slipping)…On the moon.
- Swim…In gelatin…In whipped cream.
- Stuck in a box.
- Walk the dog.
- Ride a racehorse…Bucking bull…Motorcycle.
- Hit a home run.

Variations:

1. No words can be spoken at all; only gestures and actions can be used. Have students talk about the performance after the activity is complete.

2. Students can take turns leading the activity with you prompting.

3. For extra fun and giggles, perform actions in slow motion or fast motion.

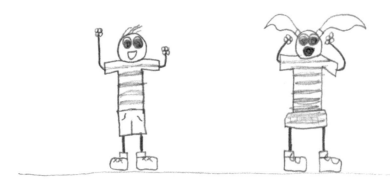

I'm a mime

Communication Link

Purpose: To learn how to give and follow clear directions effectively, use expressive and receptive language, move in unison, practice motor thinking, pretending, and problem solving.

Materials: Open space (half a room is fine).

Description: This is for children who can speak but have trouble communicating with others in terms of giving and following directions. In this exercise the main goal is to communicate effectively so that the movements work and no one falls down. The objective is to direct the group of students working as one solid line to cross a goal two to ten feet (50 centimeters to three meters) away. Have the students line up side to side with their feet touching (see illustration below). Have someone be the captain only if your students need this. Try not to give them any rules. Let them naturally elect a leader and come up with their own strategies for reaching the goal without breaking the line. This is a tricky exercise because they have to keep their feet touching their partners' feet at all times. Pretend that their feet are tied to their partners on both sides. They have to give commands in a way that won't make other students lose their balance. If the line breaks they have to go back to the initial start point and try again. The game ends after ten minutes or when all students reach the goal line.

Variations:

1. Have the children sit around in a circle after the game and talk about the strategies that worked and those that didn't work. Ask them how they felt when they weren't being heard or when others told them what to do. Tell them to talk about feelings of frustration, accomplishment, fear of falling, or anything else that they felt during the exercise. Explain that the goal of the game wasn't to finish but rather to be able to talk about the task afterward and practice solving problems.

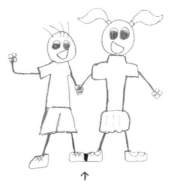

Communication link

Rhyming to the Beat

Purpose: To practice rhyming words, auditory discrimination, figurative language, slang, idioms, dancing, clapping, balancing, and singing.

Materials: Large piece of paper and markers or eraser board and dry-erase markers.

Description: Have the students (small group) line up in front of an eraser board or a large piece of paper. Have them do a beat with their feet or their hands, or, if you want, have them hold musical instruments like maracas, drums, or anything that will make noise. Once the beat gets going start them off by moving side to side to the beat or with an easy dance they can do. You want to explain to them that you are making a rap song. Take turns asking the students to make up one line of the rap until you have a full rap that you can all sing and dance to.

- Beginner: Make the rap ahead of time but leave blanks that can be filled in by the students. Printing a bunch of rhyming families works well, too, because you can cut the words out and have the students glue them on to make silly rhymes.

- Advanced: Have the students do their own rhyme and take turns performing them to their classmates or to their family.

Variations:

1. If your students cannot read you should print out pictures of rhyming families. For instance, print out pictures of a cat, a hat, a bat, a mat, and fat. They can take these pictures and place them on the rhyme. You can read the rhyme to them, but the whole class can "read" the pictures, too. Another variation is to use instruments or noisemakers to enhance the music experience.

Idiom Act-Out

Purpose: To increase awareness of idioms and figurative language and to have a good time and be silly. This activity promotes gross muscle movement and imagination.

Materials: The "Idioms List" in the Appendix.

Description: This activity will help students understand the difference between literal and figurative speech. The students are to stand loosely in a circle with you visible. You will explain, "Today we will talk about figurative and literal language. I will call out an idiom. You will act it out. That is literal language. Then I will tell you the true meaning, which is figurative language. Let's try one: 'I'm pulling your leg.'" The students will act this out. After approximately 20 to 30 seconds, interrupt and ask students for the figurative meaning: "I'm pulling your leg means what in figurative language?" The students should be given time to discuss and make attempts at the meaning. You can then give the answer if the students didn't know it: "It means, I'm teasing you." Then read another idiom and repeat the process.

Morphing Emotions

Purpose: To increase the ability to display and interpret emotions. To strengthen body awareness and muscle control.

Materials: "Table of emotions and feelings" in the Appendix. Background music never hurts.

Description: The students and you stand in a circle. Explain that you will call out an emotion (such as happy). The students are to act out and make sound effects (laugh or giggle for happy, boohoo for sad, grunt for grumpy) for that emotion (observing one another) for 30 seconds to a minute. You will then say, "Melt." The students will melt to the floor. You will call out another emotion (such as sad). The students will slowly morph into the new emotion as they rise from the floor and act it out for another 30 seconds to a minute.

Variations:

1. The students can use a mirror to monitor themselves, or if a mirror is not available they can use each other as a mirror.

2. The students can take turns calling out emotions.

3. Instead of making sound effects, students can take turns expressing why they feel a particular emotion: "I feel happy because ...." or "I feel sad because ...."

Multi-Throw

Purpose: The purpose of this activity is to improve coordination, endurance, visual perception, giving and following directions, cooperation, teamwork, sportsmanship, and pragmatic skills.

Materials: A kickball, a Frisbee™, a smaller ball (such as a tennis ball), four bases, and a bucket.

Description: The number of players recommended is 4 to 12. Have the students arrange the bases in baseball-diamond formation. Place the bucket in the middle of the field. Put the Frisbee, kickball, and tennis ball at home plate. One person is at home plate. The rest of the players are spread out around the field. The person who is up begins by throwing the Frisbee™, kicking the kickball, and throwing the tennis ball. As the student is throwing and kicking, he or she should label the object and the actions (e.g. "I am kicking the ball"). When the last ball is thrown the person who is up begins running around the bases. The students out in the field begin scrambling for the balls and the Frisbee. The object is to get the Frisbee, tennis ball, and kickball into the bucket before the runner returns to home plate. As the players are gathering up the objects they are encouraged to communicate with one another. They can say, for example, "Toss the kickball to Ryan." Once the runner makes it all the way around the bases, another runner rotates in. Students should be encouraged to use good sportsmanship and make positive comments such as "Good job," "Nice try," and "Great throw." At the end of the game, all players should shake hands and again make a positive comment or compliment.

Back to Back

Purpose: To develop interpersonal communication, coordination, teamwork, balance, and strength. Back to Back will also help students give and follow directions while not facing their communication partner.

Materials: None.

Description: Put the students into pairs of similar body weight and height. Have the students stand back to back to each other and interlock arms. The most natural way of interlocking the arms is by linking them at the elbows like hooks. Tell the students that they are now one being and that they have to coordinate their moves to prevent them from losing their balance. Ask the students to sit on the ground without letting go of their partner and remaining back to back. This may take some verbal commands from the team members to try to do it without falling. Once they have discussed possible ways of doing the task, they can go ahead and do it. After all the students are seated on the ground back to back and still interlocked with their partner, give them the next challenge—standing up again. After the challenges are finished ask some questions like, "Were you afraid that your partner wouldn't be able to hold you?" "Did you feel vulnerable at any point?" "Did you trust your partner?" "How well were you communicating?" "Did you want to listen to your partner?" and "Did any problems arise, and if so how did you solve them?" Talk about any feelings that may have arisen because of the nature of this exercise.

Variations:

1. Have the students go through different obstacles while pretending to be one person. You can have the children go through a door while still being interlocked. You can also hold a broom at chest height and have them go under it together. They must keep talking to each other to prevent failure.

Trust Walk

Purpose: To develop communication between partners, trust, use of descriptive language, coordination, balance, and walking.

Materials: Bandannas, scarves, or eye masks to cover the eyes.

Description: Have the students pair up with someone that they trust or feel comfortable with. Have one student in each pair cover his or her eyes with a bandanna or a scarf. The student will be led around by his or her partner, who holds the blindfolded student's hand and describes the path the entire time. At no point can the student who is blindfolded be left unattended or alone. The leader will say things like, "We will be taking three steps forward," "Now walk to the right," "There is a big green bush and we have to walk around it," and "Now touch this." The blindfolded student will be given things to smell and will also have to describe what he or she feels, hears, smells, and touches. Once the blindfolded student has touched or smelled at least five things the student can come back, take off the blindfold, and try to guess what he or she was touching, smelling, or hearing.

Variations:

1. You can have bowls with exotic fruits placed around the classroom (make sure you have no allergic students first). Have the leaders take their blindfolded buddies around the room to the different fruit stations. Have cut-up versions of the foods as well as whole and unpeeled versions. Some children are scared to taste anything, so be careful to assure them that everything is safe and that no one will play tricks on them. This is definitely a trust walk so they have to trust each other.

The Midas Touch

Purpose: To develop thinking, problem solving, communication, balancing, moving items without the use of hands, and carrying.

Materials: A bucket, four to five edibles, short ropes (hearty strings work, too), and sticks. Snack packs of food such as granola bars, trail-mix packets, and cracker bags work great.

Description: Read the story of King Midas and the magic touch. Explain to the students that they now have the magical powers of King Midas and that everything that they touch will turn to gold. But there is a problem. They have to bring food to a hungry friend across the room, and they are not allowed to touch the food items or the bucket directly otherwise the food will turn to gold and become inedible. The students have been given the ropes and sticks and the bucket with the food items. They have to get it all across the room to their friend, and if any food items fall out or they touch the bucket they have to start over. Try to get the students to talk to one another throughout the activity so that they can get the job done. Ask them, "How did you feel when things didn't go as well as you wanted?" "How did you deal with the feelings?" and "How did you feel when you finally got the job done?" Explore with the entire group what this exercise really taught them. How did they feel not being able to touch things?

Variations:

1. Beginners: Have the students move the bucket across the floor.

2. Intermediate: Do the activity but try not to use the floor. The bucket needs to be carried.

3. Advanced: Have the students fill the bucket using the sticks to get the food inside.

Sports Collage

Purpose: To develop fine and gross motor skills, spatial awareness, public speaking, and listening skills, and to encourage language development.

Materials: Poster board, magazines with sports-related pictures, glue sticks, and a variety of scissors.

Description: Have the students leaf through the magazines to find the desired pictures for the collage. They will cut out the pictures and talk among themselves about how they envision the collage—for example, a baseball theme or an Olympic theme. The pictures will be arranged and placed on the poster board. In this project the students work together to complete it. Each student stands up and talks about the poster and his or her contributions to it.

Variations:

1. Turn your 2D collages into 3D by rolling, flattening, shaping, and sticking pieces of play-dough onto the pictures. For example, roll a ball of play-dough and stick it to a ball in the picture, flatten it down, glue it, and let it dry. Students get to use their imagination and creativity to determine where to place the play-dough.

2. The students can make individual posters of their favourite sport or activity. When complete, the students can stand and explain their posters to each other.

3. Students can also glue seeds, small sticks, pebbles, string, tin foil, or any small objects to enhance the collage and turn it into a 3D masterpiece.

4. Collage within a shape. Have students choose a shape, related to the collage, and assemble pictures into that shape. For example, students working on a basketball collage could arrange pictures into the shape of a basketball.

Fling Sock Golf

Purpose: To develop gross motor skills, visual motor skills, group participation, topic maintenance, and vocabulary enrichment.

Materials: A fling sock for each participant. A fling sock can be made by inserting a tennis ball into a tube sock and knotting it at the end.

Description: In a group of students (this works best if the group has fewer than ten students), the players find an agreed target to fling the sock at. An example may be a pole, a bench, or a trash can. Students take turns flinging their socks toward the target. Other verbs such as *throw*, *toss*, and *pass* can be substituted for *fling* as the game progresses. The students are required to keep track of the number of throws it takes to reach the target. Once all players have reached the target the students take turns announcing how many flings they made to reach the target (e.g. "I reached the bench in five flings"). The students begin again and a new target can be selected. The targets may be distant, difficult, or easy. Players will take turns selecting and agreeing on the next target.

Variations:

1. Prior to initiating the game, students can agree on the number of targets and what they are and map out a course to follow.

2. An official scorekeeper and announcer can be chosen for each round.

3. If fling socks are not readily available, Frisbees, beanbags, rolled socks, or a ball may be used. The students can choose the item to be flung. Provide the students with the opportunity to use a ball and realize it may not be the best choice since it will bounce away from the target.

Idiom Wall

Purpose: To improve hand dexterity, manipulation of objects, fine motor movements, idioms, metaphors, and similes.

Materials: Paper and pencils, markers, or crayons.

Description: The object of this activity is to create a set of drawings that can be placed in the classroom, fridge, or student work wall so that they may create a learning board. Have the students fold the paper into four squares. Explain that they will be drawing the literal meaning of an idiom, metaphor, or simile. Give them an idiomatic expression and have them draw what they think the expression represents. For example, for the expression *Hold your horses*, the students can draw whatever they think that means. Give them about five minutes to finish their drawing. Then explain what *Hold your horses* means: "It means to calm down or slow down." When they are done give them another idiom. Do this for all four squares. Once they have finished their drawings place them on the fridge or wall with the idiom meaning on top and the drawings beneath. If you do this for a few weeks you will end up with an idiom learning tool that they will remember because they had a personal stake in it. The students feel a sense of accomplishment and they learn new words every week.

Variations:

1. Keep their drawings in a cubby or folder. After they have ten or so, staple their drawings together to create a book of idioms that they can share with their parents, friends, and relatives.

FEELINGS AND FIGURATIVE LANGUAGE

Face to Find the Place

Purpose: To learn how to read facial expressions while walking, crouching, bending, and crawling.

Materials: An object that will be used to hide.

Description: In this game the students will take turns hiding and finding an object, but the clues to finding the hiding place will be given by facial expressions. The teacher will pick one student to hide the object and another student (the finder) to go wait outside. Now explain to the class that when the finder comes back into the room the whole class has to use three facial expressions to lead the finder to the place where the object is hiding. The three expressions will be *happy* (for getting close to the object), *sad* (for getting far from the object), and *straight face* (for when the finder is equally far and close to the object). The students will not be able to use words to help the finder. Once the finder reads the cues and finds the object, he or she then gets to pick a student to give the object to and this person will be the new finder. This is a Speech in Action version of the game Hot or Cold.

Variations:

1. You can change the facial expressions to different things for a bigger challenge—for instance, *tired* for far, *excited* for close, and *confused* for equidistant. You can also use recyclable materials to make the object that will be hidden. Smaller objects about the size of a fist work best because they are relatively easy to hide.

Mining for Gold

Purpose: To develop abstract communication through map making and to strengthen muscles by walking, crouching, reaching, crawling, and bending.

Materials: Pencil, paper, spoons or shovels, rocks, and gold spray paint. If you don't have spray paint or rocks you can substitute pennies or loose coins.

Description: Take the rocks and spray paint them until they are golden. Let them dry while the students do the next part of the activity. Have them draw a map of their garden, their playground, or wherever they will be hiding their rocks. They will have to dig on the ground and make a hole where they will bury their rock. Make sure that the map includes an X where the treasure of golden rocks is found. Each student gets to decide where they will be hiding their rock and will make the appropriate map. Once all the maps have been drawn give your students a chance to go hide their rock. Then have them switch maps with somebody. If it is easier for you, collect all the maps and hand them back out, making sure no one gets his or her own map. Have the students go to the area where the gold is hidden and read their map. After everyone has found his or her rock talk about why maps are a form of communication. Explain why maps are so effective at communicating to anyone in the world, no matter what language they speak. Talk about other ways that we communicate that are universal.

Variations:

1. You can put the students in groups and have the groups look for the gold together.

2. Have students help out others once they find their rock.

Blind as a Bat

Purpose: To learn sound discrimination, walking, balancing, maneuvering obstacles, and giving and following directions.

Materials: A scarf or something to cover up the eyes; chalk.

Description: Explain how bats move. Talk about how bats have no sight but they see by hearing the world around them (sonar) and interpreting these sounds as sight. Tell the students that in this exercise they will be blindfolding one person (the bat) and he or she will have to listen to directions from one person in order to get through the obstacle course. Have all the students participate in drawing an obstacle course on the ground with the chalk. Make it wind and have things drawn on it like lakes, alligators, lions, and any other traps that the bat will have to avoid. Choose a student to be the leader and one to be the bat. The leader has to remain behind the obstacle and give verbal directions to the bat so that the bat can make it safely to the end of the obstacle course. Have everyone who feels comfortable enough to do this activity do it. If they are not comfortable being blindfolded then have them shut their eyes instead. Afterward talk about how it felt to have to rely on verbal communication in order to move. Ask the students what the hardest part of this activity was. Did they have trouble moving when they couldn't hear? Did the other students' chatter interfere with the leader's commands?

Variations:

1. You can make this activity more challenging by having two students give directions at once. Then have the whole class give directions at the same time. The student will have to learn how to discern the leader's voice from the other voices. Then talk about how noise pollution might affect our friends the bats. You can also make it more challenging by adding real obstacles, but don't use things that might be dangerous or tip over easily.

Let Me In

Purpose: To practice making requests, idioms, slang, antonyms, synonyms, cardiovascular exercises, and WH-questions (the five question words: "Where," "Who," "Why," "What," and "When").

Materials: The "Idioms list" in the Appendix.

Description: In this game the students will be in an open area where they can form a circle by holding hands. There will be one student left outside the circle (you can pick one). Give each student an idiom to memorize; they don't have to know what it means. If they have a hard time remembering you can photocopy the "Idioms list" in the Appendix and cut it into strips with one idiom per strip. They can keep it in their pocket in case they forget. The students then hold hands in a circle to form the castle walls and wait to be asked questions by the student outside the circle. The outsider has to ask questions so that he or she can find out what idiom each student is carrying. If the outsider doesn't know what the idiom means then he or she has to ask another student. This goes on until the outsider finds an idiom that he or she knows. When the outsider gets it right he or she has to ask to be let into the castle. Once let inside the castle the student gets to be king and gets to give a command. The student can say, "Run to the door, touch it, and then come back". All the students have to listen to the king and run quickly back. The last person to come back becomes the outsider and play resumes from the start.

Variations:

1. You can use antonym, synonym, or slang lists to change the game around. (See the "Antonyms list for elementary students," the "Antonyms list for middle school and high school students," the "Synonyms list," and the "Slang terms" in the Appendix.)

Place Your Guess

Purpose: To learn idiomatic expressions and manners; to develop coordination and aim; to practice bending over; and to exercise legs with sprints.

Materials: Two receptacles. A paper ball for each player (see the "Materials List" in the Appendix).

Description: Have the students make a ball out of paper or foil or something on hand. Go to an area where you can place the two receptacles ten feet (three meters) away from the students. Have them line up, facing the receptacles. Explain to them that you will be saying an idiom (from the "Idioms List" in the Appendix or your own) and then giving two definitions. The first definition will be related to receptacle A and the second definition will be related to receptacle B. They will then have to decide which definition is correct and, on your mark, run over to the receptacles to drop their paper ball inside the receptacle they chose. Let the students know which answer was correct and have them take their ball again. Try to emphasize that as long as they have a ball they have a vote. Some students will cry about wanting their personal ball back but this is a great opportunity to teach sharing and community property. Make sure they are running safely and that when they bend down to get their ball back they make sure to watch out for bumping heads. They can learn manners as well by waiting their turn, asking another student to hand them a ball, saying thank you, etc.

Variations:

1. After each idiom is defined have the students take turns aiming and throwing their ball at the appropriate receptacle. After another idiom is defined have them run the ball over to the receptacle. This gives them one turn to calm down and catch their breath again.

Line 'Em Up

Purpose: To learn figurative language, body language, and gestures while practicing reading emotions.

Materials: None.

Description: The object of this game is to get the students to line up in height order without using their voices. They have to use their bodies to "speak" and their hands to gesture directions. They will need to be very attentive to each other's faces for clues as to what their friends want them to do. They will also need to use their bodies to arrange themselves in the correct height order. Talking is absolutely not allowed. They must learn to read each other's cues. After the game is over ask them how they felt about not being able to communicate with their words. Ask them if they were frustrated and if so how they overcame their frustration. You might also want to talk about how often we use our abilities to read people's emotions on a daily basis. Why is this ability so important?

Variations:

1. For beginners have the students line up boy-girl-boy-girl.

2. For more advanced students have them line up in age order or by the year they were born. This proves to be quite fun because they have to use their fingers to "tell" one another the year they were born, and it can get quite difficult.

CHAPTER 5

The Field Trip

Some may wonder what a student with a disability may get out of going on a field trip. Let me say, every student at every level will grow and learn at least one thing from a field trip. Exposure to new experiences can broaden acceptance of new situations and places, capture and inspire special interests, hone pragmatic skills, and increase tolerance for longer or more demanding outings. It can be difficult to know how much each student understands from his or her environment, but students will often surprise you with things they pick up when no one thought they were listening. Or perhaps the best thing a student can get from a field trip is simply the experience itself.

Warning! Field trips for students with disabilities are not without difficulty. Instructors, moms, dads, and caretakers must plan field trips with care and consideration for the students. Sensory issues that may arise, such as temperature, noises, and crowds, need to be considered for a safe and positive experience. What gets students excited, or too excited? What stresses them out? What do they need to be comfortable (chew tube, fidget toys, Thomas the Tank)? If all considerations have been taken, your jaunt should be a success. If things still do not work out, and there will be times they won't, have an exit plan.

Know your students. Understand what motivates and what triggers your students prior to any outings. If your students like bubbles or music, take those items with you. If you have students who have the potential to run out into traffic, avoid high-traffic areas. Environmentally challenging locations should be avoided for students with mobility challenges. Knowing your students could mean the difference between a successful outing for both the student and the instructor and neither student nor instructor wanting to venture out again.

Previewing the day's events and scheduling outings on a regular basis will make field trips less stressful. Some students will look forward to an outing without a lot of advance information and some students like to know what to expect. Not everyone likes surprises.

Finally, know your venue. If possible scout out the area. Will it be crowded? Will there be noises? Some audio and visual stimulation can be a good thing, but too much can be bad. Check out seating arrangements and bathrooms. Is there a safe, quiet place to take a break? Is there an off-peak time to visit that is not as crowded or noisy? Knowing the area, knowing your students, preparing your students, knowing their and your limits, and having an exit plan will ensure positive, enriching experiences for all.

Trip to the Park

Purpose: To improve coordination, range of motion, body awareness, and following directions, and to increase language development.

Materials: Imagination.

Description: You will announce, "We are taking a trip to the park. When we get there we will have to ...." (you will give activities and the students follow the directions).

- Jump over ten rocks.
- Duck under three trees.
- Run from a dog.
- Talk to a baby (*ooo, eee, ba ba ba, ooo, eee*).
- Stick tongue out at a bully.
- Reach for the monkey bars.
- Spin on the merry-go-round.
- Tiptoe past a sleeping baby.
- Go swimming.

Variations:

1. Take a trip to the zoo, forest, jungle, museum, your home, etc.
2. Students take turns calling out activities to do at the park.
3. Pretend it is raining, snowing, windy, hot, and cold.

Smell the Flowers

Purpose: This activity gives the students aerobic exercise with bending, squatting, and reaching. It builds vocabulary and concept development for descriptors and adjectives using four concrete senses and one imaginary sense. Students will also be introduced to an idiom.

Materials: All that is needed for this activity is a sharp eye.

Description: You and the students go on a brisk walk in search of flowers, blossoms, pretty leaves, and grasses. When a flower is found, you will all say, "Take time to smell the roses." Each student will then smell it, touch it, see it, listen to it, and imagine what it would taste like. The students may need to bend over, stoop, squat, and reach to get access to the flowers. Do not pick or harm the flower, leaf, or grass.

- See words: pretty, red, bright, shiny, beautiful, lovely, delightful, gleaming, vibrant, colorful.

- Touch words: soft, velvety, smooth, delicate, silky, rough, prickly, coarse, jagged, slick.

- Listen words: quiet, rustling, hush, calm, still, nothing, mute, peaceful.

- Smell words: sweet, pleasant, fresh, good, bad, fragrant, aromatic, perfumed.

- Taste words (imagine): sweet, sugary, delicious, sour, bitter, spicy, tart, sharp, harsh, good, rotten.

Variations:

1. Take a sensory walk that focuses on leaves.
2. Take a sensory walk that focuses on one sense at a time.

Aquarium

Purpose: To promote the use of shape comparatives, superlative adjectives, and descriptors. The Aquarium supports large-muscle strength, facial-muscle strength, and endurance with deep knee bends, pointing, reaching, mobility, tiptoeing (reaching tall), and relaxation.

Materials: No materials required; however, books or pictures about fish would support the activity.

Description: The Aquarium field trip can be made to any neighborhood pet store or fish store. This activity can help prepare students for longer, more challenging trips. Prior to embarking on the field trip, you will review types of fish, how they breathe, and where they live (pictures and books can be utilized). Next the students can lie on the floor and pretend to be a fish moving through the water. They can make exaggerated facial expressions to simulate a fish breathing through its gills. They may also pretend to be a fish out of water and flop around until they make it back to water. Finally, the students can walk or ride to the pet store or local fish store. Once there they can look at and describe the fish according to color, size, shape, number, and personal favorite. While looking at the fish they are encouraged to bend, stretch, tiptoe, and point while describing the fish. They may take turns talking about their favorite fish. They can take notes and make drawings to construct a memory book to share with family and friends.

Variations:

1. The same activity can be utilized for a trip to the desert. The students can explore reptiles, scorpions, and lizards.

2. If the pet store has other animals then the students can pretend to take a trip to the zoo.

THE FIELD TRIP

Survey the Mall

Purpose: To develop social pragmatics, awareness of emotions, walking, asking questions, fine motor skills for holding the pencil, collecting data, and discussing results.

Materials: Clipboard and pen or pencil.

Description: Practice asking questions in class until the students feel confident. Take the students to a shopping center or a mall and ask them to pick a notetaker. The notetaker will hold the clipboard. The rest of the students will have the job of asking people who walk by a question. They will have to get the person's attention, greet the person, ask the person a question, and then thank him or her for participating. The student will then have to relay the information gathered to the notetaker. Kids really love asking questions once they get over their initial shyness. At the end of the session take the results back to the class and discuss any feelings they had toward the activity. How did they feel when they talked to strangers? How did they get over their shyness? What helped them be good surveyors? Then tally the results and post on a board or refrigerator to show off the fruits of their labor. What did we find out from the survey? Any conclusions?

Sample Questions:

What kind of ice cream do you like?

What kind of pet do you have?

Do you like dogs or cats?

Where did you go for your vacation?

What is your favorite type of soda?

Do you have any kids?

What do you like better, meat or fish?

How many hours do you sleep a night?

Do you like apples?

At what time do you go to bed?

Do you have a sweet tooth?

Have you been on a roller coaster?

What present do you want for your birthday?

If you could live anywhere where would it be?

Variations:

1. For nonverbal students write the question on a piece of paper and have them show the paper to potential participants. When they answer the question help the student find the corresponding column and tally one slash for the data collected on the clipboard.

2. For intermediate students have them ask a two- or four-answer question. For instance, they could ask, "Do you like chocolate, hard candy, lollipops, or gum?" Then as they get more advanced you can even ask an open-ended question like, "What kind of weather do you like best?"

Backyard Campout

Purpose: This activity inspires imagination, storytelling, teamwork, vocabulary building, and problem solving. It also improves muscle strength and coordination.

Materials: Old blankets, a tent (if available), flashlights, string, rope, chairs, and miscellaneous camping or pretend camping equipment.

Description: The backyard campout has been successful in many locations: backyard, living room, clinic, and office. Start this activity by announcing, "Today we are going on a camping trip." The students can choose a destination or randomly pick from a map or globe. After a destination is chosen, weather, clothing, food, and camping equipment can be discussed. The students can begin by pitching their tent or building it by tying blankets to chairs and available structures (encourages problem solving and imagination). Some students can "gather wood" while others "prepare food." Food preparation usually involves popcorn or fruit. When the wood (pretend or imaginary) is gathered and food is prepared, the students can start the campfire by rubbing sticks, fingers, or pencils together and blowing on the pretend fire to get it started. They can then all sit in a circle around a campfire (pretend) and tell stories and jokes, sing, or do skits. If inside, turn off the lights and have the students use flashlights to find their way back to their tent and go to sleep. A few minutes later they can pretend to wake up, pack up, drive home, and put the equipment away.

Variations:

1. Within this activity there are many variations depending on location, time limits, and abilities. Be open and flexible. If available and supervised, have a real fire and roast marshmallows.

2. Change from a backyard campfire to a best-friend sleepover.

Grand Central Station

Purpose: To create awareness of others and to practice manners and gross muscle coordination. This activity builds self-confidence for crowded or unfamiliar places.

Materials: None. A narrow hallway or passageway would help facilitate this activity.

Description: Students stand shoulder to shoulder in two equal lines facing each other, approximately ten feet (three meters) apart. Instruct them to walk toward each other. When they get approximately an arm's length away they do not stop walking but say, "Excuse me," "Pardon me," "Coming through," or "Can I get by?" They then turn sideways and pass by each other (remembering to give eye contact and a smile). You will then reinforce the importance of eye contact and a smile and practice again. When the students have mastered this activity, you can take them into the crowded halls for a real-life practice session. You will be amazed at how social students become in crowded situations and by the positive reactions from peers.

Variations:

1. When the students are ready, take them to a crowded store or restaurant or mall for more real-life practice.

2. This activity also works for introductions. Instead of excusing themselves and moving through a crowded group, have the students stop and introduce themselves first, make a comment, and then move on.

Trip to the Store

Purpose: This activity promotes bending, stretching, helping, following directions, asking questions, and identification of items by attributes. This activity also gives students an opportunity to practice manners and social pragmatics.

Materials: No materials needed. A shopping cart or basket can be used if desired. If only a few items are to be purchased, have students carry unbreakable items to keeps hands busy and increase sensory input.

Description: Prepare the students for the store by making a list of items needed. Each student can have his or her own list or they can all have the same list. They can write, type, draw, or have pictures of needed items. Walk to the store if possible. Upon entry to the store, one student is to hold the door and the others should say thank you as they pass. One student can push a basket (for breakables) and the others can carry unbreakable items. While shopping the leader will ask a student to reach for the yellow can of corn or the blue bag of chips. The leader can ask for several items from the top shelves so that the students can stretch. If the item is not needed then the leader simply says, "Oops, didn't need that. Can you put it back?" This gives the students plenty of stretches and keeps them busy. The same technique can be done for items on the bottom shelf. The leader can say, "Can you bend down and get the small bag of flour?" If the leader did not really need the flour then say, "Oops, my mistake. Can you put it back?" Once again, this gives the students extra opportunities for bending and stretching (as in the illustration below).

Variations:

1. Leaders can be rotated as they finish their lists or part of a list.

2. Leaders can incorporate numbers and sensory details (smooth, slushy, ripe smell, sour).

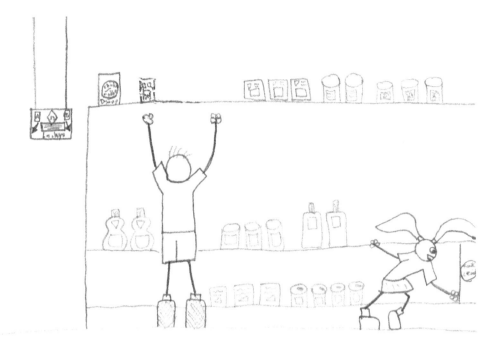

Trip to the store: Stretching and bending

125

Walking: Corner Talk

Purpose: To improve sense of direction, communication, agility, and motor skills. To strengthen vocabulary and describing skills.

Materials: Gym, school ground, park, or community area.

Description: Have the group of students walk to the corner. Once they reach the corner, have them describe what they see (people, places, and things). When each student is finished with the description, walk to the next corner. Repeat the descriptions.

Variations:

1. Once all of the descriptions of the corners have been made, the students can retrace the walk. For example, one student might say, "Walk to the corner with the vine." The group walks to the corner where the vine is growing. Another student might say, "Walk to the corner with two trash cans," and the group follows.

2. You can also use walking variations for this part of the activity. For example, one student might say, "Shuffle to the corner with the bench. Skip to the corner with the trash can."

3. After the walk, sit and review from memory what each student saw.

Jump

Purpose: This activity increases large-muscle strength, muscle grading, and fine-muscle coordination. It increases body awareness, identification, and community labeling.

Materials: No materials needed, but you can string a line across the room and hang various items (clothes, paper, shapes, napkins, placemats, etc.) at various heights to fit the students' abilities.

Description: Announce that everyone is going on a jumping walk. At this point, you should demonstrate and have the students practice jumping over items and jumping up to touch items. When the opportunity presents itself, have the students jump and touch leaves, branches, a sign, or an overhang. You can say, "Jump for the leaves" or "Jump and touch the biggest leaf with your thumb." If there is a curb available you can have the students jump up or down the curb (if safe). Look in the environment for things to jump over or up to touch. Encourage the students to look for opportunities to jump. They can take turns being the leader and calling out opportunities to jump. Students usually are very creative in calling out scenarios and will generalize this activity in family walks.

Variations:

1. This activity can be done in a gym or large room using a string to hang items.

2. The students can have a friendly competition by determining who can touch the highest leaf or jump over the most cracks in the sidewalk. You should encourage and model good sportsmanship.

Trip to an Orchard

Purpose: To develop the use of descriptive language, coordination, balance, walking. To answer WH-questions, retell a story, and expand on events.

Materials: Money to buy a few fruits. Plastic cutlery and plates.

Description: Have the students go up and down ladders, if available, to reach the fruit in the orchard's trees. Let them pick the fruit and tell you why they chose the fruit that they picked. What were their criteria? Did they use the same criteria for all the choices? Then walk around the orchard. Walking on rugged terrain with rocks, sticks, and fallen fruit will raise their awareness, especially when they walk on soft soil that gives a little. This walk will require a lot of balancing and coordination because of all the obstacles they will have to walk around. As they are walking have them talk about the sights, sounds, smells, and sensations they encounter. Once finished they can bring their fruit back to the school or eat it there under a tree in a picnic-style lunch.

Variations:

1. Make a fruit salad with the different things that the students picked. They can practice their cutting with the plastic knives. Discuss the attributes of the fruit and the experience. Have them retell their favorite part of the trip. Ask who, what, when, where, why, and how questions so that they can recall important details about the trip.

I Spy Safety Signs

Purpose: To increase safety awareness and knowledge and comprehension of the purpose of signs. To practice reading safety signs. This is also a walking activity that increases general physical fitness and stamina.

Materials: None needed. However, if the students have the ability to write they can bring clipboards and keep track of the signs by writing or drawing them on paper. Pictures of safety signs to support the activity, if available.

Description: Begin by explaining what safety signs are and why they are important. At that point, the students can practice stopping, walking, waiting, and going one way. When the walk begins, you will say, "I spy the safety sign stop." All participants should walk to the sign, read it (sign or picture exchange), and write it down. Then they can all practice stopping by walking to the sign and stopping several times. Prompt the students to begin looking for another safety sign by saying "I spy a safety sign _____" and looking around. When another sign is spied, the student should say, "I spy the safety sign _____." All participants will walk to that sign, write or draw it, and act it out several times. The length of the walk will depend on students' abilities and endurance.

Variations:

1. All community signs can be read, written, or drawn, and acted out (if appropriate).

2. Signs such as "Open," "Closed," "Hours," and "Discounts" on businesses can be explored.

3. The students can make social stories or storyboards from their drawings and writings.

4. This activity can also be fun in a mall if the weather is too hot or too cold outside.

CHAPTER 6

Success Stories

Earl

Earl was my most challenging student and the student who set me on the path to *Speech in Action*. He was a nonverbal teenage boy who frequently had aggressions when asked to participate in a task (therapy, vocational, or academic). Earl had many years of discrete trial and tabletop therapy to increase his communication skills. He was capable of utilizing a picture-exchange system; however, he chose not to. I had never thought about incorporating movement into my sessions until the day I saw Earl having a great time participating and completing tasks for the adaptive physical education (APE) specialist. Earl not only completed all tasks but he was happy and laughed on more than one occasion. Hmm. The next session I asked the APE specialist if I could incorporate some language goals into Earl's physical education routines. It worked! After a few sessions, Earl was attempting vocalizations, utilizing his picture exchange, and making gestures more frequently than ever before. Today, Earl still does not enjoy tabletop structured activities; however, he is able to request movement breaks and does his tasks to earn trips to the movement room. Aggressions have gone down in the classroom and I am able to achieve my communication goals in positive, productive sessions. My first success!

Gaston

Gaston is an 18-year-old highly verbal student. He is constantly on the move and frequently paces in the back of the classroom. Traditional sit-down-and-focus learning environments are difficult for him. Too much of Gaston's valuable therapy time was utilized in keeping him at the table or in a chair. Language-movement groups that focused on figurative language and pragmatic skills were a perfect fit for him. Now he is able to spend his entire therapy time focusing on goals in a structured, purposeful movement environment. Today Gaston is a teacher's assistant for the movement groups. He has learned leadership and negotiation skills well. His vocational goal is to be an adaptive physical education assistant. At his Individual Education Plan meeting Gaston reported to the entire team, "I can't learn unless I am moving." Success!

Fiona

Fiona is a beautiful 14-year-old who is nonverbal with fleeting eye contact. At home and in the classroom she frequently has negative behaviors when she is stressed. I started working with her in the movement room when I noticed she enjoyed the swing and scooter. I soon realized that she was making eye contact and attempting to communicate when movement was part of the routine. After a couple of weeks of language-movement sessions, she would make eye contact and emit a "haaa" sound. On week three we began our session. Fiona excitedly sat down with the group. She made eye contact with me and started vocalizing the haaa sound. After several attempts of haaa, the sound clearly emerged into a "Hi." Today, Fiona continues to expand her ability to communicate with vocalizations, picture exchange, and gestures. Her demeanor is happy and her parents report she has generalized both movement and communication skills into the home. Success!

Danielle

Danielle is a student with autism. She is 12 years old, has strong receptive-language skills, and loves dancing and riding bikes. She had been participating in traditional speech therapy for many, many years. Danielle traditionally speaks in single-word utterances if at all. I started working with her utilizing movement to strengthen expressive language. It worked! Somehow the movement and getting caught up in the moment increases her words per utterance. She is generally happier and teachers and caregivers are now utilizing the same strategies to increase expressive language at home and in the classroom. One morning while riding on the adaptable bike, it appeared that the seat was too high. I asked her if she wanted me to lower the seat. She responded to me, "The seat's fine." We proceeded to ride about the campus. After a 15-minute ride, I said that it was time to go back to the gym. Danielle kicked up the pedaling and raced down to the gym. She came within a few inches of the wall and made a skillful turn away from the wall. This was followed by a professionally maneuvered S turn, and she impressively guided the bike through a narrow doorway. Danielle performed one more lap around the gym before coming to a stop. She pulled off her helmet and announced, "I finished the obstacle course." Success!

APPENDIX

Table of body parts

ankle	arm
back	belly
calf (plural: calves)	cheek
chin	ear
elbow	eye
eyebrow	eyelash, lash
finger	fist
foot (plural: feet)	forehead
hair	hand
head	hip
knee	leg
lip	lower leg
mouth	neck
nose	shoulder
thigh	thumb
toe	tongue
tooth (plural: teeth)	underarm, forearm
waist	wrist

Table of emotions and feelings

absurd	adventurous	affectionate	afraid
aggravated	agitated	agreeable	alone
amused	angry	animated	annoyed
anxious	appreciation	apprehensive	argumentative
astounded	awkward	bewildered	bitter
blessed	blissful	bored	bothered
brave	bright	bursting	calm
captivated	careless	caring	celebrating
charmed	cheerful	cold	comfortable
compassion	concerned	confused	cool
creative	cross	delighted	depressed
discomfort	disgust	disturbed	doldrums
dull	eager	ecstatic	enchanted
endearing	enjoy	enraged	enthusiastic
exasperated	excited	fear	flattering
flustered	fretful	frustrated	fun
furious	fussy	giggly	glad
gleeful	gloomy	good	grateful
grief	gusto	harsh	hectic
hilarious	hopeful	horrified	humorous
hysterical	impressed	impulsive	infuriated
interested	intimidated	intrigued	irritated
jealous	jolly	joy	lethargic
light hearted	lonely	lonesome	love
mad	melancholy	melodramatic	merry
miserable	mopy	nervous	nonchalant
optimistic	panic	passive	patient
perky	pity	pleasant	proud
quiet	reckless	refreshed	ridiculous
safe	satisfaction	scared	secure
seething	selfish	serious	shame
shocked	shy	silly	sincere
stressed	stunned	suffer	sweet
sympathy	thrilled	tickled	timid
uncomfortable	unhappy	warmhearted	weary
welcomed	whiney	worried	zealous

APPENDIX

135

Table of occupations

accountant	actor/actress	acupuncturist	administrator
ambassador	anchorman	animal trainer	archaeologist
architect	artist	astronaut	athlete
attorney	babysitter	baker	bank teller
barber	biologist	blacksmith	bookkeeper
brain surgeon	cab driver	cardiologist	carpenter
cartoonist	cashier	chef	chemist
chiropractor	coast guard	comedian	construction worker
cook	dancer	dentist	deputy
dermatologist	detective	disc jockey	doctor
editor	electrician	engineer	explorer
farmer	firefighter	fisherman	florist
game warden	gardener	governor	grocer
hairdresser	hairstylist	handyman	ice cream man
illustrator	inventor	janitor	jeweler
journalist	judge	landlord	lawyer
lifeguard	locksmith	magician	maid
mailman	marine biologist	mayor	mechanic
model	musician	nanny	nurse
occupational therapist	optometrist	orthodontist	painter
paramedic	pediatrician	pharmacist	photographer
physical therapist	physiologist	pilot	plumber
police officer	president	prime minister	professor
publisher	reporter	rockstar	sailor
salesman	scientist	sheriff officer	shoemaker
singer	speech therapist	spy	surgeon
taxi driver	teacher	veterinarian	watch maker
weatherman	writer	zookeeper	zoologist

American Sign Language alphabet

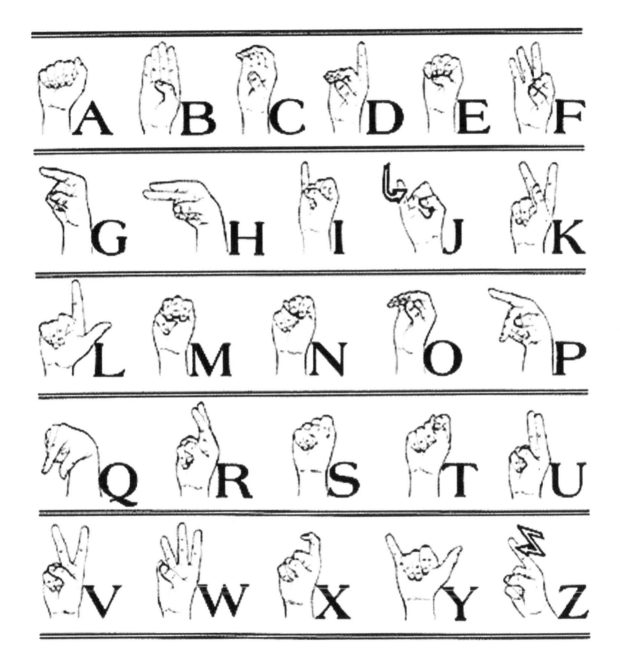

Reproduced with permission from Martin Frost.

Synonyms list

alternative—option

caution—care

copy—duplicate

damp—wet

distribute—dispense

fight—battle

gaze—stare

hate—dislike

hurry—rush

liberty—freedom

lump—chunk

neighborhood—community

paw—foot

poison—toxin

prison—penitentiary

sad—unhappy

stay—wait

substitute—replacement

tow—pull

veer—swerve

big—large

center—middle

courageous—valiant

danger—hazard

divide—separate

fire—blaze

get—receive

hear—listen

inappropriate—improper

lid—cover

mission—assignment

odd—strange

petty—unimportant

ponder—contemplate

quick—fast

small—little

stop—halt

sudden—unexpected

traditional—customary

weaken—undermine

categorize—classify

clench—squeeze

crash—smash

disappear—vanish

exaggerate—magnify

funny—amusing

harm—hurt

hesitant—indecisive

inspect—examine

lost—missing

natural—organic

paste—glue

pick—choose

present—gift

restriction—limitation

smile—grin

stream—creek

tough—rugged

unprotected—vulnerable

Antonyms list for elementary students

add—subtract
all—none
begin—end
big—small
brave—cowardly
come—go
cute—ugly
diet—binge
east—west
empty—full
fat—thin
front—back
guilty—innocent
honest—dishonest
inside—outside
least—most
long—short
man—woman
night—day
old—young
over—under
positive—negative
quit—persevere
rich—poor
safe—dangerous
sick—well
stop—go
top—bottom
whisper—shout
yes—no

after—before
always—never
below—above
black—white
bright—dull
correct—incorrect
cut—paste
dirty—clean
easy—difficult
far—near
find—lose
give—take
hard—soft
hot—cold
last—first
light—dark
loud—quiet
mean—kind
normal—abnormal
open—close
patient—impatient
punish—reward
reject—accept
right—left
same—different
silence—noise
strong—weak
up—down
wide—narrow

alive—dead
asleep—awake
best—worst
boy—girl
ceiling—floor
create—destroy
daughter—son
done—start
eat—fast
fast—slow
forward—backward
good—bad
hit—miss
ill—well
laugh—cry
light—heavy
love—hate
more—less
off—on
out—in
pleasant—unpleasant
push—pull
remember—forget
sad—happy
shallow—deep
sit—stand
tall—short
wet—dry
work—play

Antonyms list for middle school and high school students

abandon—pursue
abuse—praise
adamant—flexible
admit—deny
always—never
attic—cellar
banish—summon
believe—question
bizarre—common
bony—boneless
busy—idle
cheerful—depressed
close—far
collect—distribute
compare—contrast
concrete—abstract
cursed—blessed
defeat—victory
destroy—create
down—up
eccentric—typical
existence—nonexistence
extract—insert
finite—infinite
forward—reverse
frozen—melted
gracious—impolite
great—small
homogeneous—
heterogeneous
imitation—original
inhale—exhale
joined—disconnected
just—unjust or unfair
kill—give birth to
late—early
loud—quiet
marry—divorce

abandon—restraint
accept—refuse
adept—inept
adorable—repulsive
appear—disappear
attractive—repulsive
bashful—bold
beneficial—harmful
bland—spicy
brash—cautious
capitalist—socialist
cheer—jeer
coastal—inland
combined—separated
competent—incompetent
connected—disconnected
darkened—brightened
deny—admit
detached—attached
dull—bright
enter—exit
expanded—concise
faceted—faceless
fix—break
free—confined
gentle—harsh
gradual—sudden
hairy—bald
hospitable—inhospitable

immediate—slow
intense—mild
joyful—melancholy
keep—give
kiln—freezer
leading—following
love—hate
masculine—feminine

above—below
achieve—fail
admirable—despicable
alive—dead
asleep—awake
bald—hairy
beginning—end
big-wig—Joe-schmoe
bona fide—fake or unreal
brave—cowardly
careful—careless
clear—opaque
cold—hot
compact—loose
concave—convex
crystalline—cloudy
decrease—increase
desecrated—consecrated
distributed—concentrated
eager—reluctant
equal—unequal
expensive—affordable
fail—succeed
forward—backward
frequent—seldom
geriatric—neonatal
grainy—smooth
hide—reveal
hydrophobic—hydrophilic

impartial—biased
intentional—accidental
junk—precious
key—unimportant
last—first
life—death
malignant—benign
matter—antimatter

meager—ample
monochromatic—polychromatic
near—far
nothing—everything
omnipotent—powerless
pass—fail
positive—negative

pristine—dirty
provincial—cosmopolitan
question—answer
rainforest—desert
reported—censored
rush—dawdle
self-centered—altruistic
stormy—calm
tantalizing—uninviting
terrestrial—aquatic or aerial
transmissible—incommunicable
uncomfortable—comfortable
vacant—occupied
vibrant—spiritless
weathered—new
worst—best
yes—no
zany—humorless

midnight—midday
multiplication—division

nonchalant—concerned
objective—subjective
opposite—same
passive—active
posterior—anterior

productive—unproductive
public—private
quick—slow
raw—cooked
repulsive—attractive
scarce—abundant
serene—agitated
subtraction—addition
tarnished—stainless
tight—loose
unaware—alert

undercooked—burnt
valiant—cowardly or wimpy
villain—hero
whole—fractional
wrong—correct
yours—mine
zig-zag—straight

mixed—pure
natural—unnatural

northern—southern
occidental—oriental
outrageous—inoffensive
past—future
postmeridian (pm)—antemeridian (am)

progress—regress
quaint—familiar
quiet—loud
real—unreal or fake
resentful—forgiving
scream—whisper
single—multiple
superior—inferior
temporary—eternal
timid—bold
unchanged—altered

unsure—confident
vanish—appear
weak—strong
wise—foolish
yell—whisper
youthful—aged
zipper—button

Idioms list

Idioms marked (UK) are used predominantly in British English; those marked (AUS) predominantly in Australian English.

A
acid test
act of God
add fuel to the fire
afraid of your own shadow
against the clock
all ears
all fingers and thumbs
all hands on deck
all the rage
ants in your pants (UK)
apple of someone's eye
as easy as pie
as flash as a rat with a gold tooth (AUS)
as the crow flies (UK)
at arm's length
at the eleventh hour

B
back to square one
backseat driver
bad egg
bad hair day
bad-mouth (verb)
bait and switch
ball and chain
(the) ball is in your court
bark up the wrong tree
beat about the bush (UK)
beat around the bush
beat your brains out
bee in your bonnet (UK)
belt and braces (UK)
bent out of shape
between the devil and the deep blue sea (UK)
beyond the black stump (AUS)
bite off more than you can chew

blow your top
Bob's your uncle! (UK)
bold as brass (UK)
brass-monkey weather (UK)
Break a leg!
break someone's heart
break the ice (UK)
bull-headed
burn the candle at both ends
burn the midnight oil
butter someone up
by the skin of your teeth

C
call it a day
call your bluff
can of worms
can't make head or tail of
carrot and stick
cash in your chips
catch 22
catch red-handed
catch some rays
catch some Zs
catch your eye
(the) cat's pajamas
chicken out
cheap as chips (UK)
chip off the old block
chow down
(to be) cool
Cool it!
cost a bundle
cost an arm and a leg
couch potato
Cut it out!
cut down the tall poppies (AUS)
(the) cutting edge

D
damp squib (UK)
dangle over their head
dead as a doornail
devil's advocate
different kettle of fish
dig in your heels
do a bang-up job
do someone's dirty work
do the running (UK)
done up like a dish of fish (UK, AUS)
down in the dumps
drag one's feet

E
(to be an) eager beaver
earn a crust
Easy does it!
elbow grease
Excuse my French! (UK)

F
fair crack at the whip (UK)
Fair dinkum! (AUS)
fall on deaf ears
fed up (with)
feel blue
fire someone
fly off the handle
follow your heart
food for thought
force of habit
forty winks
free as a bird
free ride
free-for-all
fresh as a daisy
frog in your throat
front runner
full of hot air

G

gather dust
Get a grip!
get a kick out of something
get cracking
get off someone's back
get off your high horse
get on your nerves
get out of hand
get the nod (UK)
get up and go
get your act together
get your ducks in a row
get your wires crossed
gift of the gab
give someone a hand
give someone the red carpet treatment
go over your head
go with the flow
grab a bite
grasp the nettle (UK)

H

hammer it out
handle with kid gloves
hang in there
happy as a clam
happy-go-lucky
Hard cheese! (UK)
have a ball
have a heart
have your hands full
head honcho
hit the hay
hit the sack
hold the baby (UK)

I

icing on the cake
in a tick (UK)
in over your head
in spades (UK)
in the bag
in the black
in the dark
in the red
in the same boat
industrial-strength

J

jack of all trades
jaw-dropping
jog your memory
join the club
jump to a conclusion
(the) jury is still out
just what the doctor ordered

K

keen as mustard (UK)
keep an eye out for
keep in touch
keep it together
keep it under wraps
keep your chin up
keep your fingers crossed
keep your hair on (UK)
keep your nose to the grindstone
keep your options open
keep your pecker up (UK)
kick your heels (UK)
kick yourself
know something inside out

L

labor of love
lame duck
land on your feet
lash out
last straw
laughing stock
lay down the law
leave no stone unturned
left to your own devices
leg it (UK)
lend a hand
(a) lick and a promise (UK)
(a) little bird told me (UK)
low blow

M

mad as a cut snake (AUS)
made of money
make a beeline for something
make a mountain out of a molehill
make a song and dance about something (UK)
make ends meet
make or break
make up your mind
make waves
make your blood boil
meet me halfway
milk it
miss the boat
money doesn't grow on trees
money to burn
month of Sundays (UK)
mug's game (UK)
Mum's the word! (UK)

N

nailing jelly to the wall
name is mud
neck and neck
needle in a haystack
nerves of steel
next to nothing
no hard feelings
No way!
not cricket (UK)
Not on your life!

O

off color
off the cuff
off the record
old wives' tale
oldest trick in the book
olive branch
on the back burner
on the back foot (UK)
on the ball
on the cards (UK)

143

on the dot
on the go
on the road
on the trot (UK)
on thin ice
once in a blue moon
out of pocket (UK, AUS)
out of the blue

P
packed like sardines
pain in the neck
paint the town red
paint yourself into a corner
paper trail
partner in crime
pass the buck
pay peanuts
pay the piper
peas in a pod
piece of cake
pull someone's leg
pull your finger out (UK)
put your foot in your mouth

Q
quick as a fox
quick fix
quiet as a mouse

R
race against the clock
rack your brains
rain or shine
raining cats and dogs
raise eyebrows
rake over the coals
rant and rave
reach for the moon
read someone's mind
red tape
rip off
rise to the occasion
rub someone the wrong way
rude awakening

S
save your breath
saved by the bell
scare someone to death
scratch the surface
sea legs
second nature
see which way the cat jumps (AUS)
sell your soul
set in stone
She'll be apples. (AUS)
shoot the breeze
sleep on it
sooner or later
spin a yarn (UK)
state of the art
Step on it!
sticky wicket (UK)
stiff upper lip (UK)
Stone the crows! (UK, AUS)

T
take a backseat
take a load off
take a nosedive
take it easy
take someone to the cleaners
take someone under your wing
take the bull by the horns
take the floor
talk the hind legs off a donkey (UK)
talk the legs off an iron pot (AUS)
talk to the hand
taste of your own medicine
tight with money
tight-fisted
thin edge of the wedge (UK)
to your heart's content
tough luck
two-faced

U
ugly duckling
under the weather
under your belt
until hell freezes over
until you're blue in the face
up a gum tree (AUS)
up and running
up for grabs
up in the air
uphill battle
upper hand
use your noodle

V
vanish into thin air
vertically challenged
vicious circle

W
waiting in the wings
walk on air
walk on eggshells
watch like a hawk
watch your step
weak in the knees
wear many hats
wear out your welcome
wear the pants
wet behind the ears
white lie
with bells on

Y
yes-man
Your guess is as good as mine.
Your blood is worth bottling. (AUS)

Z
zip it
zone out

Slang terms

A
ace (UK)—excellent; great
aggro (UK)—(short for aggravation) = violence
airhead—dumb person
anorak (UK)—geek
arvo (AUS)—afternoon
Aussie—Australian
awesome—great; impressive

B
bangers (UK)—sausages
bang—powerful effect
barbie (UK, AUS)—barbecue; grill
barmy (UK)—foolish; mad
beans—money
beast—savage person
beat—tired
beemer—a BMW
biccie (UK)—biscuit
biggie—something important
biker (UK)—motorcycle rider
bird (UK)—woman; girl; girlfriend
bitzer (AUS)—mongrel dog (bits of this and bits of that!)
blag (UK)—robbery
bloke (UK)—man
bod—body
bonkers (UK)—crazy
bonzer (AUS)—great
booboo—mistake
bread (UK)—money
brew (UK)—tea or coffee
brill (UK)—abbreviation of brilliant
buck—dollar

bunk off (UK)—be absent without permission
bushed—extremely tired

C
cakehole (UK)—mouth
cheesy—lacking in good taste, unstylish
chicken—coward
chook (AUS)—chicken
chuck up—vomit
cool—excellent; superb
couch potato—person who watches too much television
cozzie (UK, AUS)—swimming costume
cranky—in a bad mood; angry
crikey (UK, AUS)—expression of astonishment
cushy—easy

D
dead cert (UK, AUS)—something definite
deck—knock down
dicey—unpredictable; risky
ding-dong (UK)—argument; fight
dinosaur—something out of date or old-fashioned
doddle (UK)—something easy
dodgy (UK, AUS)—dubious (person or thing)
doobry—a nonsensical word used when you forget the name of something

dork—dumb or inept person
dosh (UK)—money
down under (UK)—Australia and New Zealand
dude—man
dynamite—powerful; excellent

E
earbashing (UK, AUS)—nagging; nonstop chatter
eyeball—stare long and hard at

F
fab (UK)—short for fabulous
face-off—confrontation
fender-bender—minor car accident
five-finger discount (UK)—shoplifting
flaky—unpredictable
flummox—confuse
footie (UK)—(short for football) = soccer
freebie—something that does not cost money
full-on—powerful; with maximum effort
funny farm—mental hospital or institution
funny money—counterfeit money

G
geek—eccentric person or misfit, often with an obsessive interest in something
get it—understand

go ballistic—go crazy with anger

go bananas—go crazy

good on ya! (AUS)—good for you! well done!

goof off—waste time

goof—silly person

grand—one thousand dollars or pounds

grubby—dirty

grub—food

grungy—dirty and/or in poor condition

guts—courage

H

hacked off (UK)—fed up, annoyed

hairy—difficult; dangerous

ham-fisted (UK)—clumsy

have a gander at (UK)—look at

headcase (UK)—crazy person

hip— fashionable

hole in the wall (UK)—ATM

hoop-la—trouble; commotion

hot—popular; attractive

hottie—attractive person

huff (UK)—bad mood

humungous (UK)—really big

I

icky—unpleasant

iffy—dubious, doubtful

ivories—teeth

J

jammy (UK)—lucky

jerk—dumb or annoying person

jock—someone good at sports

K

kick back—relax

kip (UK)—sleep

knackered (UK)—exhausted

knock back (UK, AUS)—refuse, turn down

knockout—beautiful woman; handsome man

kook—peculiar strange or eccentric person

L

laid back—relaxed; calm

lairy (UK, AUS)—loud, brash

lame—weak; unfashionable

lip (UK)—cheeky talk

loaded—very rich

loo (UK)—toilet

loser—worthless person

love handles—excess fat around the waist

M

malarkey (UK)—nonsense

mate (UK, AUS)—friend

mega—big

megabucks—large amount of money

mickey-mouse—unimportant

mozzie—mosquito

mug (UK)—gullible person

N

neat—cool, great

nick (UK)—steal

nipper (UK)—small child

no-hoper (UK)—someone who'll never do well

nosh (UK)—food

not all there (UK)—stupid; crazy

nuke—cook something in the microwave oven

nutcase (UK)—odd or crazy person

nuts (UK)—crazy

P

pad—home, house

party animal—someone who loves parties

paws—hands

peanuts—very little money

pig out—eat too much

pooped—exhausted

pressie (UK)—present, gift

psycho—crazy person

R

rabbit (UK)—talk a lot

rat—despicable person

ripper (AUS)—great, fantastic

rocking—great, excellent

rubbish (UK)— nonsense

rug rat—child

rug—wig

S

scoff—eat

screw up—make a mistake

shades—sunglasses

skosh—a little bit

snookered (UK)—stuck

specs (UK)—eyeglasses

split—leave

spunky (UK, AUS)—spirited, full of life

street smart—knowledgeable about city life

sunnies (UK)—sunglasses

sweet (UK)—excellent, cool

T

tacky— lacking in good taste, unstylish

take a sickie (UK)—take the day off sick from work when you're perfectly healthy

telly (UK)—television

thingo (AUS)— whatsit, something you don't know the name of!

threads—clothing

turkey—failure, flop

turn-off—something that repulses someone

U

umpteen (UK)—countless

uptight—nervous, anxious

V

veg out—relax in front of the TV

W

wad—a lot of money

wheels—(a) car (b) motorcycle

whiz—someone who shows a special talent for something

wicked—excellent

wimp—timid or cowardly person

wuss—coward

Y

yabber (AUS)—talk

Yank—American person

yob (UK)—rowdy or aggressive young man

Z

zero—unimportant person

zilch—nothing

zip—(a) nothing (b) energy, vigor

zit—pimple

Table of descriptors

abnormal	abrasive	abusive	adorable	alluring	aloof
arrogant	aware	awesome	awful	bad	beautiful
better	black	bloated	bold	broad	broken
bumpy	busy	callous	calm	concerned	cool
courageous	crazy	creative	creepy	critical	cute
damp	dangerous	defiant	destructive	disastrous	discreet
dizzy	drab	dumb	dusty	eager	early
educated	effective	egotistical	enchanted	enormous	exclusive
exotic	expensive	fabulous	fair	famous	fancy
fantastic	fast	fat	fearful	freaky	frightened
gaudy	gaunt	gentle	giant	giddy	gifted
glamorous	grateful	great	great	handsome	handy
hard	hard	hard	harmonious	harsh	harsh
hateful	healthy	icy	idiotic	ignorant	ill
illegal	imaginary	immense	immense	imminent	impolite
jaded	jagged	jealous	jittery	jobless	jolly
joyous	juicy	jumbled	jumpy	kaput	keen
kind	kindhearted	kindly	knotty	knowing	knowledgeable
known	lacking	lame	large	last	late
lavish	lazy	light	loose	macho	magenta
magical	malicious	massive	mean	meek	messy
moody	naive	narrow	nasty	naughty	near
neat	negligent	new	nutty	obedient	obese
obscene	odd	offbeat	old	opposite	organized
overt	painful	painful	pale	panicky	peaceful
perfect	petite	pink	purple	quaint	quarrelsome
questionable	questionable	quick	quickest	quiet	quirky
quixotic	rainy	rare	rare	real	red
red	reflective	repulsive	reserved	sad	salty
sassy	savory	scared	scrawny	secret	shy
silver	tacky	tan	tart	tasty	tearful
tender	tiny	tired	tough	ugly	unable
uneven	unique	unkind	vacuous	vague	valuable
victorious	violent	vivacious	warm	wary	watery
weak	wealthy	weary	white	yellow	young
youthful	yummy	zany	zealous	zesty	zippy

"Hokey Pokey" lyrics

You put your right foot in
You put your right foot out
You put your right foot in
And you shake it all about.
You do the Hokey Pokey
And you turn yourself around
That's what it's all about.

You put your left foot in
You put your left foot out
You put your left foot in
And you shake it all about.
You do the Hokey Pokey
And you turn yourself around
That's what it's all about.

You put your right hand in
You put your right hand out
You put your right hand in
And you shake it all about.
You do the Hokey Pokey
And you turn yourself around
That's what it's all about.

You put your left hand in
You put your left hand out
You put your left hand in
And you shake it all about.
You do the Hokey Pokey
And you turn yourself around
That's what it's all about.

You put your right shoulder in
You put your right shoulder out
You put your right shoulder in
And you shake it all about.
You do the Hokey Pokey
And you turn yourself around
That's what it's all about.

You put your left shoulder in
You put your left shoulder out
You put your left shoulder in
And you shake it all about.
You do the Hokey Pokey
And you turn yourself around
That's what it's all about.

You put your right hip in
You put your right hip out
You put your right hip in
And you shake it all about.
You do the Hokey Pokey
And you turn yourself around
That's what it's all about.

You put your left hip in
You put your left hip out
You put your left hip in
And you shake it all about.
You do the Hokey Pokey
And you turn yourself around
That's what it's all about.

You put your whole self in
You put your whole self out
You put your whole self in
And you shake it all about.
You do the Hokey Pokey
And you turn yourself around
That's what it's all about.

"Dem Bones" lyrics

The foot bone connected to the leg bone
The leg bone connected to the knee bone
The knee bone connected to the thigh bone
The thigh bone connected to the back bone
The back bone connected to the neck bone
The neck bone connected to the head bone

Dem bones, dem bones gonna walk a-roun'
Dem bones, dem bones gonna walk a-roun'
Dem bones, dem bones gonna walk a-roun'

The head bone connected to the neck bone
The neck bone connected to the back bone
The back bone connected to the thigh bone
The thigh bone connected to the knee bone
The knee bone connected to the leg bone
The leg bone connected to the foot bone

Body parts and corresponding bones ("Hokey Pokey" and "Dem Bones")

ankle bone—talus
arm bones—humerus (upper); radius and ulna (lower)
back bone—spine
chest bone-—sternum
collar bone—clavicle
finger bones—phalanges
foot bones—tarsals and metatarsals
hand bones—carpals and metacarpals
head bone—skull/cranium
heel bone—calcaneus
hip bone—innominate
jaw bone—mandible
knee cap—patella
leg bones—femur (upper); tibia and fibula (lower)
neck bone—spine
ribs—costals
shoulder blades—scapulas
tail bone—coccyx
toe bones—metatarsals

List of materials

Any of the materials in the list may be used for the following equipment:

Ball materials:
crumpled paper
crumpled aluminum foil
balloon
gumball machine bouncer
wiffle ball
playground ball
sock roll

Targets:
industrial bucket
pickle barrel
packing box
stack of plastic cups

Hoops:
Hula-hoops
PVC pipe
garden hose

Collapsible targets:
milk cartons
soda bottles
tin or aluminum cans
plastic cups

Bases:
paper plates
pizza circles
cardboard squares

Bottle catchers:
half-gallon bleach bottles
large juice containers

Field markers:
half-gallon soda bottles.
tall cups
cones
rocks or bricks
milk cartons

All of the materials in the list are required for the following equipment:

Fling sock:
  tennis or hand-held ball
  tube sock

Dancing ribbon:
  12 inch (30 cm) dowels
  plastic tubing
  8 foot (2.5 m) ribbon
  colorful thread
  swivel hooks
  eye screws

Beanbag:
  any heavy duty material cut in the preferred shape
  industrial rice bags
  beans or rice

Sponge target:
  household sponges cut into 2 inch (5 cm) squares
  traditional chalk board
  sidewalk chalk
  concrete surface if the chalk board is not available

GLOSSARY

Adaptive Physical Education (APE)—an individual program of developmental activities, games, sports, and rhythms suited to the interests, capacities, and limitations of students with disabilities who cannot safely or successfully engage in unrestricted participation in the vigorous activities of the general population.

agility—the ability to change the body's position efficiently. It requires the integration of isolated movement skills using a combination of balance, coordination, speed, reflexes, strength, endurance, and stamina.

appropriate—acceptable within a given setting.

articulation—the act or manner of producing a speech sound.

body awareness—an element that comprises focus on body shapes, body base, body part, and locomotor and nonlocomotor movements.

body language—a form of nonverbal communication consisting of body pose, gestures, and eye movements. Humans send and interpret such signals both consciously and subconsciously.

communication—the process of transferring information from one entity to another.

comparatives—special form of adjectives. They are used to compare two or more things and are formed using an **-er** suffix or by placing "more" before the adjective.

coordination—the combination of body movements created with the kinematic (such as spatial direction) and kinetic (force) parameters that result in intended actions. Such movements usually work together smoothly and efficiently. Motor coordination can occur between subsequent parts of the same movement and the movements of several limbs. Motor coordination involves the integration of processes ranging from how muscles interact with the skeletal system to neural processes controlling them both in the spine and in the brain.

descriptor—a word or combination of words that can be used to describe or identify something, someone, or someplace.

disability—any impairment (physical or mental) that can make routine tasks more difficult or impossible.

endurance—the ability of the body to keep up an exercise or activity continually over a period of time without getting tired. The more endurance someone has, the longer they can swim, bike, run, or play a sport before tiring out.

expressive language—the ability to communicate wants and needs or make oneself understood, usually via speech, sign, picture communication, or writing.

figurative language—a way of expressing ideas in nonliteral or "plain" form. It can be used to add color or intensity to a description. Metaphors, similes, and idioms are examples.

fine motor—involving the small muscles of the hands, as in handwriting, cutting, or dressing.

generalization—the application of a skill learned in one situation to a different but similar situation.

gesture—a motion of the body as a means of communication or expression.

grasping—a motion of seizing, snatching, or clutching.

gross motor—involving the large muscles of the body, as in walking, running, or swimming.

idiom—a phrase or expression that is (usually) not taken literally. For example, "Don't let the cat out of the bag" means to not tell something one knows, and to instead keep silent.

inappropriate—unacceptable within a given setting.

infuse—introduce a certain modifying element, activity, or quality: "the team's continued success is attributable to a steady infusion of language acquisition and movement."

locomotor—of a self-powered motion by which a person changes their location through walking, running, jumping, crawling, swimming, or skipping.

manners—polite social behavior or skills.

metaphor—an implied comparison that brings together two dissimilar objects, persons, or ideas. A metaphor often directly identifies an obscure or difficult subject with another that is easier to understand.

mobility—movement that involves changing the position of oneself or an object. A person with a mobility impairment may have difficulty with walking, standing, lifting, climbing stairs, carrying, balancing, or having the stamina and endurance to do these kinds of activities.

motor—describing the contraction of muscles in an orderly and meaningful manner.

oral motor—of the muscle movements of oral structures (lips, tongue, cheeks, palate) during speech and feeding.

phoneme—the smallest segmental unit of sound used to form meaning.

picture exchange—the use of pictures to communicate wants, needs, requests, and thoughts.

pragmatics—the rules or practices regarding how language is used, in particular social situations, to convey social information, such as the relative status or power of the speaker.

preposition—a word used to show the relation of a noun (or pronoun) to another word in a sentence. e.g. about, above, across, after, against, along, amid, among, around, at, before, behind, below, beneath, beside, besides, between, beyond, by, down, except, for, from, in, into, of, off, on, until, unto, up, etc.

problem solving—using existing knowledge to determine the best solution to a problem.

prompt—something that indicates when or where a response is appropriate (noun). To lead someone toward what they should say or do (verb); e.g. to show or tell an actor/person the words they should be saying, or actions they should be doing.

proprioceptive—relating to the awareness of posture, movement, and changes in equilibrium and the knowledge of position, weight, and resistance of objects in relation to the body.

range of motion—the amount of movement a limb has in a specific direction.

receptive language—the understanding of speech sounds, sentences, grammatical structures, and implications of what is communicated.

self-esteem—the way you feel about yourself, who you are, the way you act, and how you look.

self-regulate—the individual's ability to recognize, direct, and modulate his or her own thoughts, feelings, and behavior without outside controls.

sensory integration—the neurological process that organizes sensation from one's own body and the environment, thus making it possible to use the body effectively within the environment. Our senses give us information about the physical conditions of our body and the environment around us. The brain must organize all of these sensations if a person is to move and learn and behave normally.

sequencing—a serial arrangement in which things follow in logical order or a recurrent pattern.

sign language—language expressed by visible hand gestures, hand shapes, facial expressions, and movements used to communicate.

simile—a figure of speech comparing two unlike things, often introduced with the words "like" or "as."

spatial awareness—the awareness of one's body and the things around it in space.

spatial relations—defines the relationship between objects. Spatial relations include qualities like size, distance, volume, order, and time. They can be between oneself and an object, like a chair, or between two objects, like a chair and a table.

Speech Language Pathologist—the professional who assesses, diagnoses, treats, and helps to prevent disorders related to speech, language, cognitive-communication, voice, swallowing, and fluency. Sometimes called speech therapists.

superlatives—special form of adjectives. They are used to compare two or more things and are formed using an **–est** suffix or by placing "the most" before the adjective.

task analysis—the breaking down of a target behavior into smaller, more manageable steps.

visual motor integration—the ability of the eyes and hands to work together efficiently for a desired outcome.

visual perception—the brain's ability to interpret and make sense of visual images seen by the eyes.

visual supports—pictures, written words, story boards, stories, or anything visual that helps the individual increase his or her understanding of language.

REFERENCES AND FURTHER READING

References

Auxter, D., Huettig, C., Pyfer, J., Roth, K., and Zittel, L. (2009) *Principles and Methods of Adapted Physical Education and Recreation* (11th edition). New York: McGraw-Hill.

Brewer, C. and Campbell, D. (1991) *Rhythms of Learning: Creative Tools for Developing Lifelong Skills.* Tucson, AZ: Zephyr Press.

Bureau of Labor Statistics (2010) 'Speech-language pathologists.' *Occupational Outlook Handbook, 2010–11 edition.* Available at www.bls.gov/oco/ocos099.htm, accessed on September 6 2010.

Connor-Kuntz, F.J. and Dummer, G.M. (1996) 'Teaching across the curriculum: Language-enriched physical education for preschool children.' *Adapted Physical Activity Quarterly 13*, 3, 302–315.

DiCarlo, C., Banajee, M., and Stricklin, S. (2000) 'Circle time: Embedding augmentative communication into routine activities.' *Young Exceptional Children 3*, 18–26.

Gould, D. (1987) 'Promoting Positive Sport Experiences for Children.' In J.R. May and M.J. Asken (eds) *Sport Psychology: The Psychological Health of the Athlete.* New York: PMA Publishing.

Hannaford, C. (1995) *Smart Moves: Why Learning Is Not All in Your Head* (2nd edition). Arlington, VA: Great Ocean Publishers.

Herman, G.N. and Kirschenbaum, R.J. (1990) 'Movement arts and nonverbal communication.' *The Gifted Child Today 13*, 20–22.

Hill, T. and Reed, K. (1990) 'Promoting social competence at preschool: The implementation of a co-operative games programme.' *Early Child Development and Care 59*, 1, 11–20.

Jensen, E. (2000) *Brain-Based Learning.* San Diego, CA: The Brain Store Inc.

Jobling, A., Birji-Babul, N., and Nichols, D. (2006) 'Children with Down syndrome: Discovering the joy of movement.' *Journal of Physical Education, Recreation and Dance 77*, 6, 34–38.

Kovar, S.K., Combs, C.A., Campbell, K., Napper-Owen, G., and Worrell, V.J. (2007) *Elementary Classroom Teachers as Movement Educators* (2nd edition). Boston: McGraw-Hill.

Mutrie, N. (1998) 'Physical activity and its link with mental, social and moral health in young people.' Young and Active Symposium, January 1 1998. Lecture conducted from Health Education Authority, London.

Waugh, L.M., Bowers, S.T. and French, R. (2007) 'Using picture cards in integrated physical education.' *Strategies 20*, 4, 18–20.

Zittel, L.L. (2005) 'Early Childhood Adapted Physical Education.' In J.P. Winnick (ed.) *Adapted Physical Education and Sport* (4th edition). Champaign, IL: Human Kinetics.

Further reading

Aitken, J.E. (undated) Greeley, CO: University of Northern Colorado. Available at www.unco.edu/AE-Extra/2008/8/aitken.html, accessed on May 30 2010.

Blinde, E. and McClug, L. (1997) 'Enhancing the physical and social self through recreational activity.' *Adapted Physical Activity Quarterly 14*, 327–344.

Chretien, K. and Miller, A. (2007) *The Miller Method: Developing the Capacities of Children on the Autism Spectrum* (1st edition). London: Jessica Kingsley Publishers.

Decker, J.I. and Mize, M.G. (2001) *Walking Games and Activities* (1st edition). Champaign, IL: Human Kinetics.

Dennison, P.E. and Dennison, G.E. (1992) *Brain Gym: Simple Activities for Whole Brain Learning (Orange)*. Ventura, CA: Edu-Kinesthetics, Inc.

Minton, S. (2003) 'Using movement to teach academics: An outline for success (movement literacy).' *Journal of Physical Education, Recreation and Dance 74*, 2, 36–40.

Murata, N. (2003) 'Language augmentation strategies in physical education.' *Journal of Physical Education, Recreation and Dance 74*, 3, 1–70.

Moving and Learning

www.movingandlearning.com

PE Central: The Web Site for Health and Physical Education Teachers

www.pecentral.org

Milton Keynes UK
Ingram Content Group UK Ltd.
UKHW030637161024
449562UK00002B/9